THE PA BIBLE

A PANCE Workbook Written by the Physician Assistants Who Wish They'd Had It

PART 1

Christine Nelson,
Tiffany Lee,
&
Meredith Allen

The PA Bible: A PANCE Workbook Written by the Physician Assistants Who Wish They'd Had It

PART 1

NELSON, CHRISTINE, Author
THE PA BIBLE
CHRISTINE NELSON

In Association with:
ELITE ONLINE PUBLISHING
63 East 11400 South #230
Sandy, UT 84070
EliteOnlinePublishing.com

ISBN: 978-1-971310-05-3 (Paperback)
MED058210
MED086000

QUANTITY PURCHASES: Schools, companies, professional groups, clubs,
and other organizations may qualify for special terms when ordering quantities of this title. For information, email
info@ eliteonlinepublishing.com.

Why We Created This Workbook

Our hope is that PA students can have most everything needed to study for the PANCE in one place, this workbook. While studying for the PANCE ourselves we spent hundreds of dollars on different books and online systems and felt overwhelmed by the options and at times too much information. We wanted to create a workbook that was directly tailored to the PANCE blueprint, user-friendly, and concise enough as to not be overwhelming. This workbook is specifically designed to categorize necessary information while allowing the student to participate in the process by filling in the information, which has been proven to help with recall and retention.

How to Use This Workbook

- We recognize some of the topics fit into multiple subjects, but we kept it simple by only putting each topic in one place in the workbook. You can find each topic in the appendix if it isn't where you instinctively think it would be.
- Some topics may not have enough room to put everything in that you learn. We recommend putting in the information that is harder to remember, and not writing what you already know. This will help to ensure that your individual workbook doesn't become overcrowded or busy.
- There are "empty" boxes within the workbook that are intended for the reader to draw or fill in that information, again this helps with recollection and learning.
- There is a section at the end of each chapter to put the most commonly used medications within each subject.
- There are also lined pages at the end of each subject so that you can add any subjects or information that you feel are important but that aren't specifically on the PANCE blueprint.

Table of Contents

Cardiology 1

Pulmonology 54

Gastrointestinal Disorders 89

Musculoskeletal/Ortho/Rheumatology 132

EENT 203

Appendix 240

Cardiology

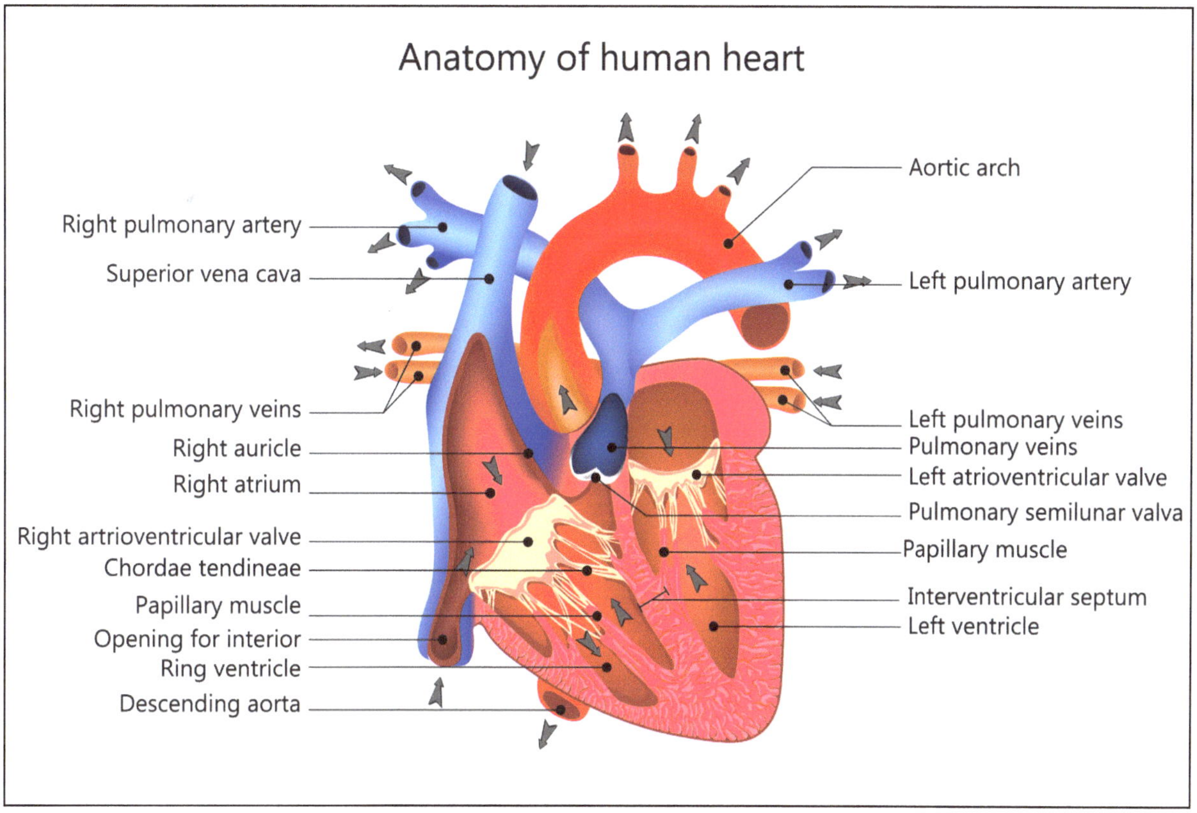

Anatomy of human heart
Right pulmonary artery
Superior vena cava
Right pulmonary veins
Right auricle
Right atrium
Right artrioventricular valve
Chordae tendineae
Papillary muscle
Opening for interior
Ring ventricle
Descending aorta
Aortic arch
Left pulmonary artery
Left pulmonary veins
Pulmonary veins
Left atrioventricular valve
Pulmonary semilunar valva
Papillary muscle
Interventricular septum
Left ventricle

Inflammatory Cardiac Disorders

Pericarditis: Most common viral (coxsackie), autoimmune

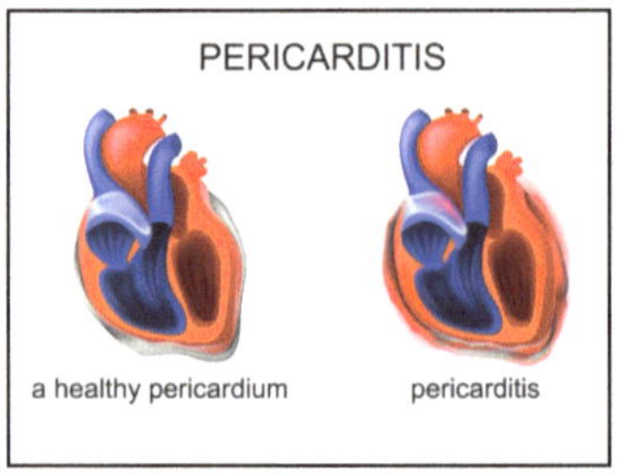

Sx:

PE: Pericardial friction rub, squeaking sound on auscultation

Dx: Serum troponin, echocardiogram, Chest X-ray, and EKG showing diffuse ST elevation

Tx:

Dressler's Syndrome: Immune response to damaged heart muscle (type of pericarditis)

Sx:

PE:

Dx: CBC shows increased WBC, CRP, & ESR

Tx:

Pericardial Effusion: Fluid in pericardial space - can lead to cardiac tamponade

Sx:

PE: Tachycardia, tachypnea, hypotension, elevated jugular venous pressure

Dx:

Tx:

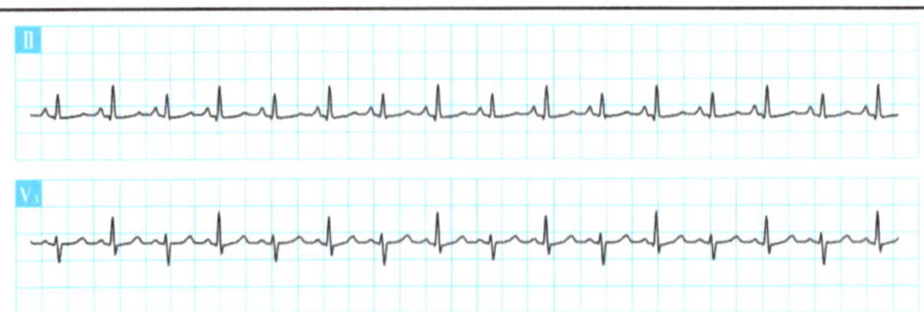

QRS wave electric alternation

QRS wave amplitude and shape alternately

Cardiac Tamponade: **Compression of all heart chambers resulting in narrow pulse pressure, pulsus paradoxus**

Sx:

PE: BECKS TRIAD =

Dx: Transthoracic echocardiogram, Chest X-ray, CBC, cardiac enzymes

____ Tx:

____

____

Myocarditis: **Cardiac muscle inflammation - can lead to CHF**

Causes: Cocaine use, post viral illness in young patients = parvovirus/coxsackie

Sx:

PE:

Dx: Elevated cardiac enzymes

____ Tx:

____

____

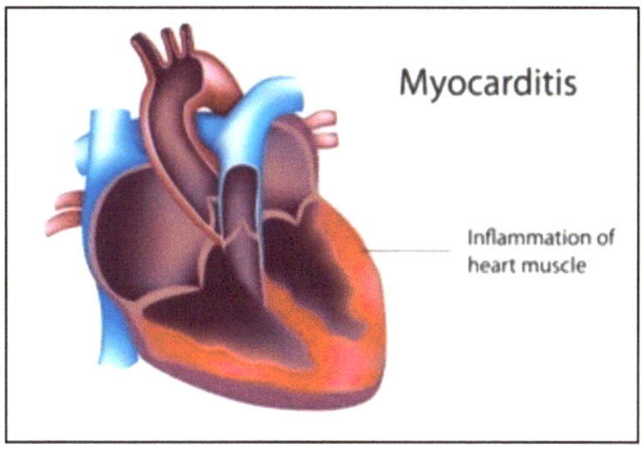

Endocarditis: Fever + new murmur

IV drug use = S. aureus (affects tricuspid)

GI cancer = Strep bovis or gallolyticus

Sx: Fever, anorexia, Roth Spots, Osler Nodes, murmur, Janeway Lesions, anemia, splinter hemorrhages

PE:

Dx: CBC, echocardiogram, EKG, blood cultures

Tx:

____

____

____

Dukes Criteria

Major Criteria:

Minor Criteria:

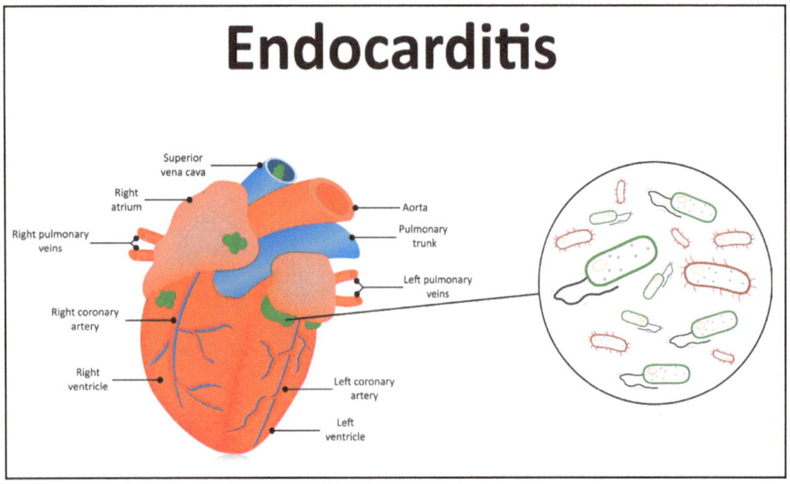

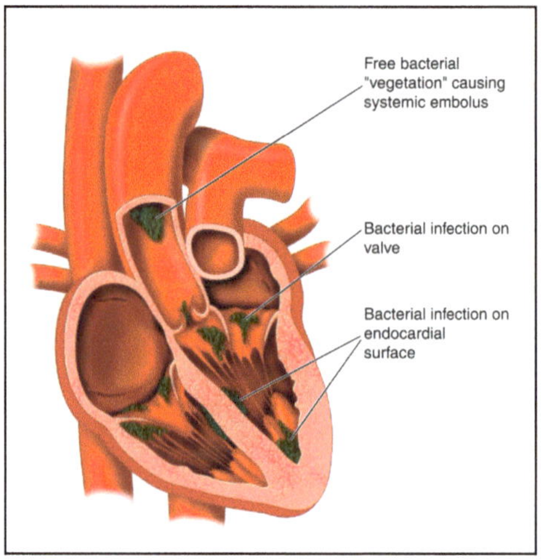

Valvular Disorders

Aortic Stenosis:

Causes: Congenital bicuspid, rheumatic fever, age, calcifications

Sx:

Murmur:

Dx: Transthoracic echocardiogram, EKG, Chest X-ray

______________________________________ **Tx:**

____

____

Aortic Regurgitation:

Causes: Marfan's Syndrome, rheumatic fever, aortic dilation

Sx: Depends on severity and cause

Murmur:

Dx:

______________________________________ **Tx:**

____

____

Mitral Stenosis:

Causes: Rheumatic fever

Sx:

Murmur:

Dx: Transthoracic echocardiogram, EKG, Chest X-ray

______________________________ **Tx:**

____

____

Mitral Regurgitation (Acute and Chronic):

Acute = sudden volume overload, acute pulmonary edema

Causes: mitral valve prolapse, ischemia

Sx: Dyspnea with exertion, lower extremity edema, fatigue

Murmur:

Dx:

______________________________ **Tx:**

____

____

Mitral Valve Prolapse:

Risk Factors: Connective tissue disorders

Sx:

Murmur:

Dx: Transthoracic echocardiogram & transesophageal echocardiogram

______________________________ **Tx:**

____

____

Pulmonary Stenosis: Can lead to right heart failure

Sx:

Murmur:

Dx: Echocardiogram

Tx:

Pulmonary Regurgitation:

Sx:

Murmur:

Dx: Echocardiogram

Tx:

Tricuspid Stenosis:

Causes: Rheumatic fever, IV drug use

Sx:

Murmur:

Dx: Echocardiogram

Tx:

Tricuspid Regurgitation: **Can be asymptomatic**

Cause: IV drug use

Sx:

Murmur:

Dx: Echocardiogram

Tx:

Rheumatic Fever: **Strep**

Sx: Jones Criteria

PE:

Dx:

Tx:

Jones Criteria	
Major Criteria	Minor Criteria

Systolic Murmurs

Diastolic Murmurs

Innocent Murmur:

Sx:

PE:

Dx: Echocardiogram with color doppler

Stills Murmurs (Type of Innocent Murmur):

Sx: Asymptomatic

PE:

Dx:

Cervical Venous Hum (Type of Innocent Murmur):

Sx: Asymptomatic

PE:

Dx: Echocardiogram

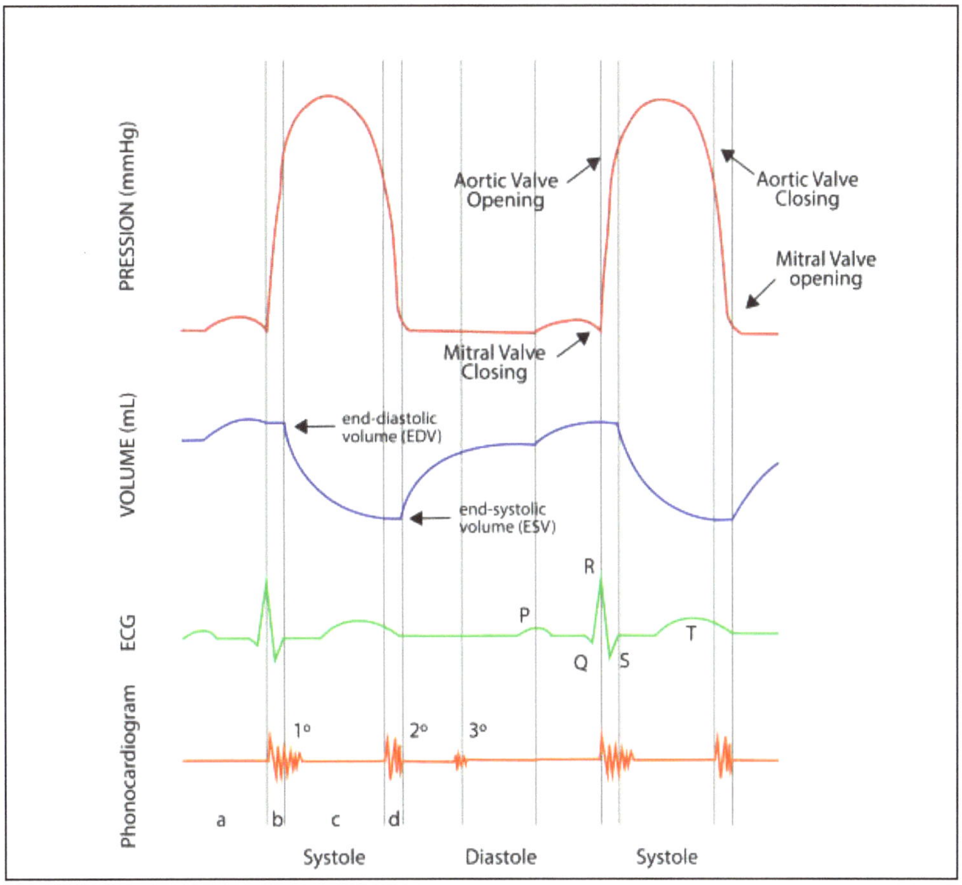

Murmur Vocabulary

Carvallo's sign = murmurs are louder with inhalation

Stenosis = not able to fully open

S1 = closure of Mitral & Tricuspid valves

S2 = closure of Atrial & Pulmonic valves

S3 = ventricular overload (rapid filling)

S4 = decreased LV wall compliance (atrial contraction)

Splitting = asynchrony between AV or semilunar valves

Click = abrupt halting of valve - leaflet folding into the atrium & suddenly stopped by chordae tendinea

Thrill = palpable murmur - feels like a vibration

Heave = abnormally large beating of the heart - sign of LVH

Diaphragm = increased pitched sounds (normal heart sounds & systolic murmurs)

Bell = decreased pitched sounds (S3, S4, diastolic murmurs, bruits)

Acute Coronary Syndrome

Stable Angina:

Risk Factors: Smoking, hypertension, diabetes, obesity

Sx: Pain with exertion that resolves with rest

PE:

Dx: Exercise stress test, EKG, HbA1c, normal troponin, & CK-MB

Tx:

Unstable Angina:

Risk Factors: Smoking, hypertension, diabetes, obesity, hyperlipidemia

Sx: Pain at rest, may not be relieved with nitroglycerin

PE:

Dx: Normal cardiac enzymes, EKG, Chest X-ray, coronary angiography

Tx:

Prinzmetal Angina: Coronary spasms

Risk Factors: Smoking, young

Sx: Mostly in the morning time

PE:

Dx: EKG with ST elevations, coronary angiography

Tx:

NSTEMI:

Sx:

PE:

Dx: Elevated troponin and CK–MB, EKG = ST depression

Tx:

STEMI:

Sx:

PE:

Dx: EKG = ST elevation

Tx:

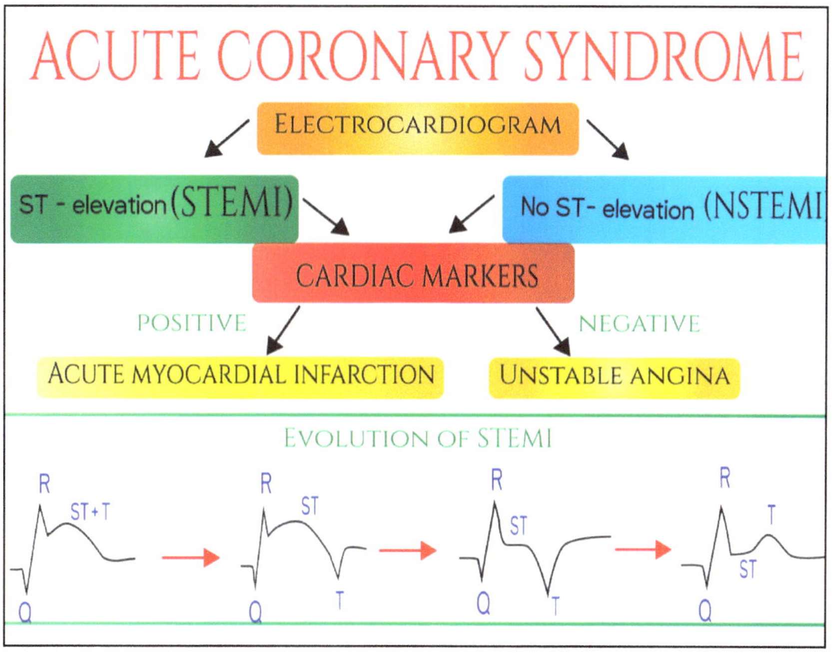

Acute Myocardial Infarction

Anterior MI

Tx:

Inferior & Right Ventricle MI

Do not use nitroglycerin, morphine, or Viagra

Tx:

Lateral MI

Tx:

Posterior MI

Tx:

Beck's Triad = decreased BP, clear lungs, JVD

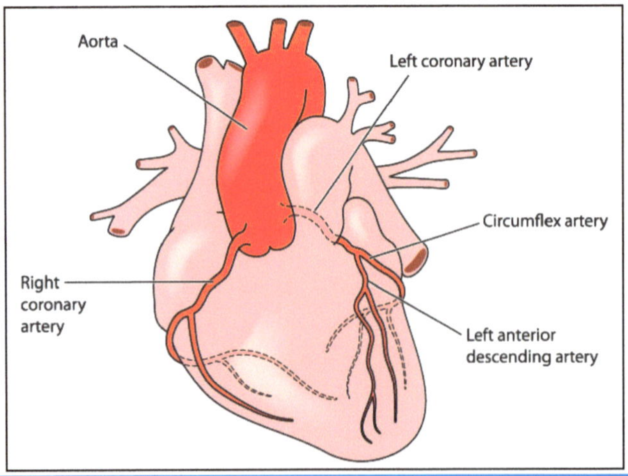

Post MI Care

Aspirin 81 mg QD (clopidogrel if allergy)

ACEI or ARB - to improve left ventricular ejection fraction

BB - decreased mortality by decreased O2 demand

- **Prolong diastole to improve coronary flow**
- **Decreased chance for V-fib**
- ***Avoid with: Bronchospasm, hypotensive & unstable, Heart block > 1st degree, heart failure***

Fiber

Statins - stabilize plaques

- **LDL < 70**

Combined aspirin/clopidogrel - use 6-12 months in stented pts

Lifestyle changes = quit tobacco, increase dietary fiber, decrease saturated fat, increase weight loss

Cardiac Rehab = medically monitored cardiovascular exercise

- **Stimulated angiogenesis**
- **Decreased post-MI depression**

Dysrhythmias & Conduction Disorders

1st Degree Heart Block: Delay @ AV node

Dx: EKG = PR interval > 0.2

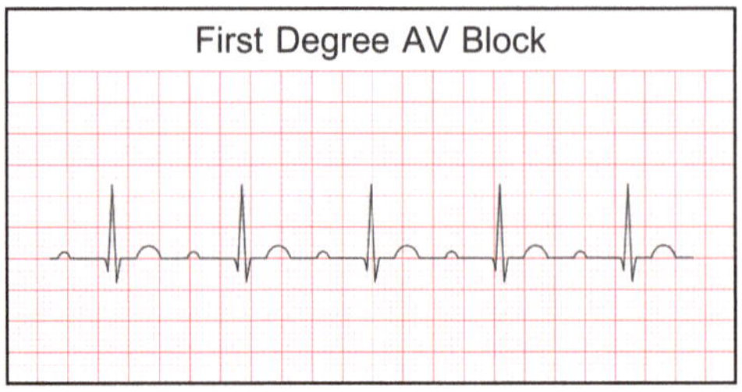
First Degree AV Block

Tx:

2nd Degree Heart Block: Mobitz I, Wenckebach

Dx: EKG = PR interval longer each cycle then drops

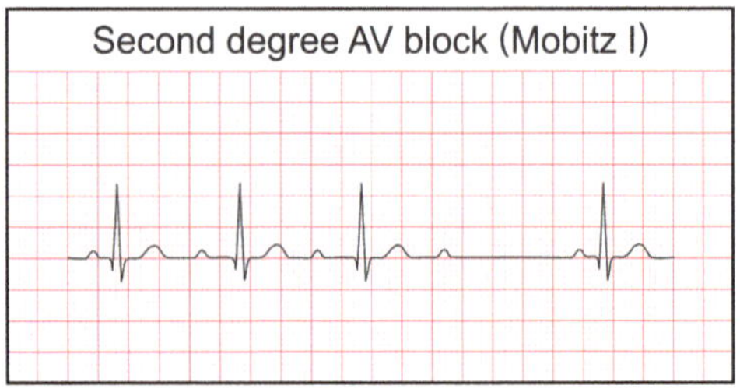
Second degree AV block (Mobitz I)

Tx:

2nd Degree Heart Block: Mobitz II - not benign - conduction system disease below Bundle of HIS

Dx: EKG = normal or long PR with dropped QRS

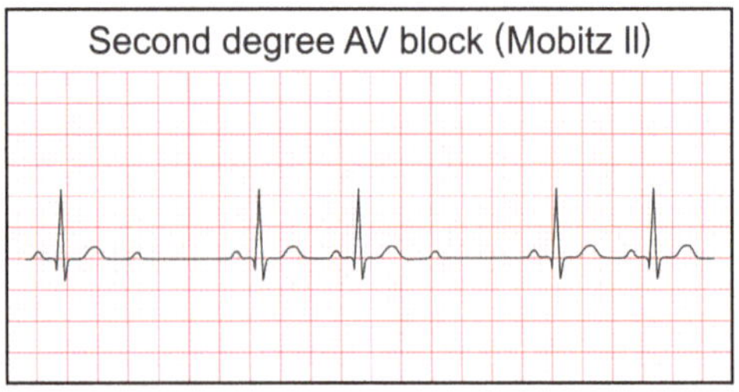
Second degree AV block (Mobitz II)

Tx:

3rd Degree Heart Block: Complete heart block - severe bradycardia due to absence of AV node conduction

Dx: EKG = independent atrial and ventricular rhythms with widened QRS complex

Cannon A wave =

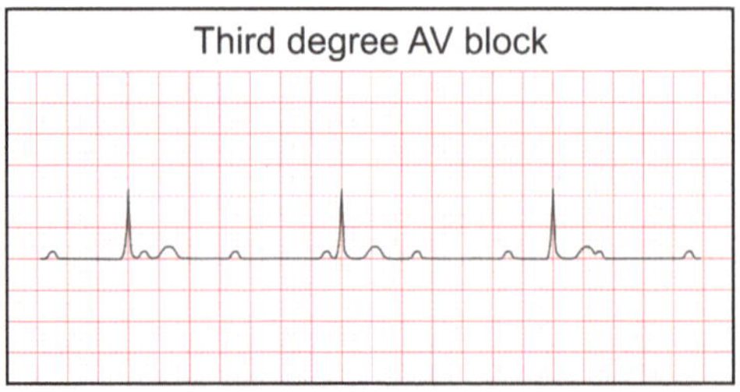
Third degree AV block

Tx:

BUNDLE BRANCH BLOCK: Often asymptomatic - ventricular depolarization takes longer

Right Bundle Branch Block: Rule out pulmonary embolism

Bunny ears in pre-cordial leads

Slurred S waves in lateral leads

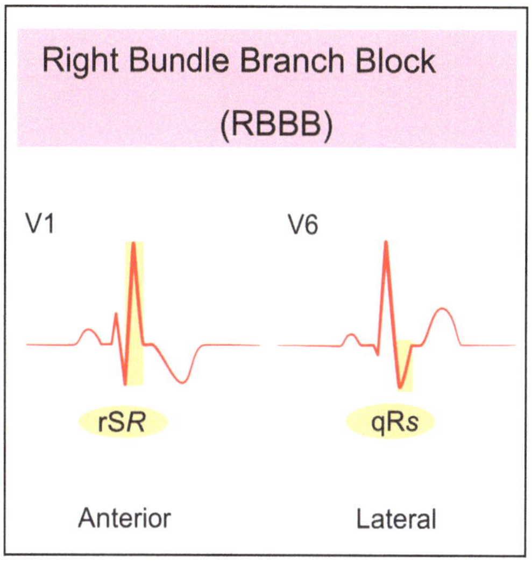

Dx:

Tx:

Left Bundle Branch Block: Rule out myocardial infarction

Absence of Q wave in lead 1, V5, & V6

Monomorphic R wave displaced opposite QRS complex

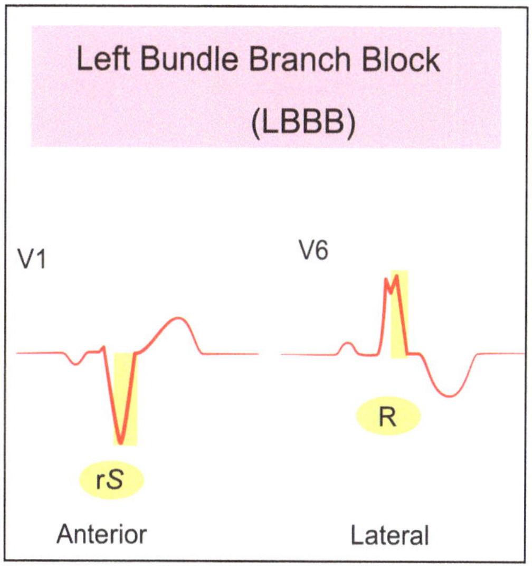

Dx:

Tx:

Sick Sinus Syndrome: Sinoatrial node dysfunction

Sx:

PE:

Dx: EKG = bradycardia, sinus pause, sinus arrest

Tx:

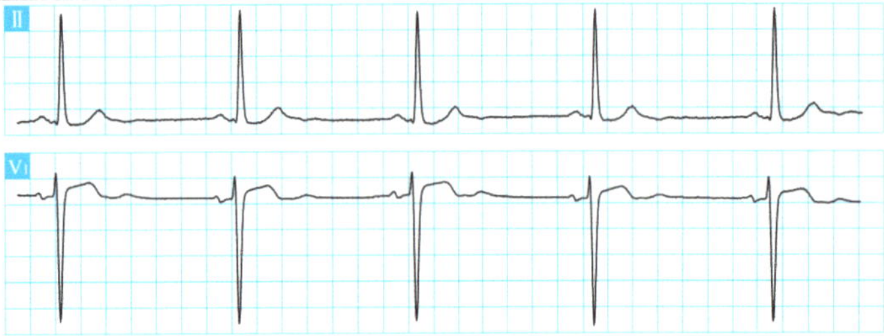

Sick sinus syndrome

Severe sinus bradycardia

Premature Beats

Premature Atrial Contraction (PAC)

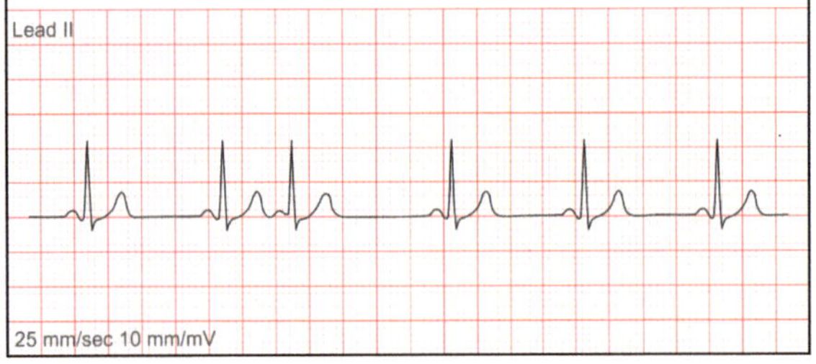

Tx:

Premature Ventricular Contraction (PVC)

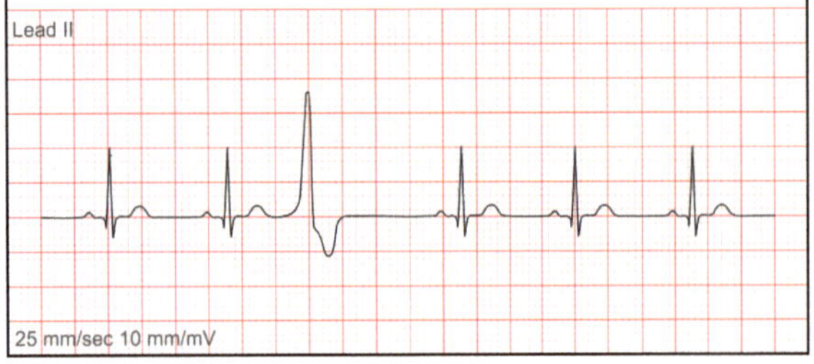

Tx:

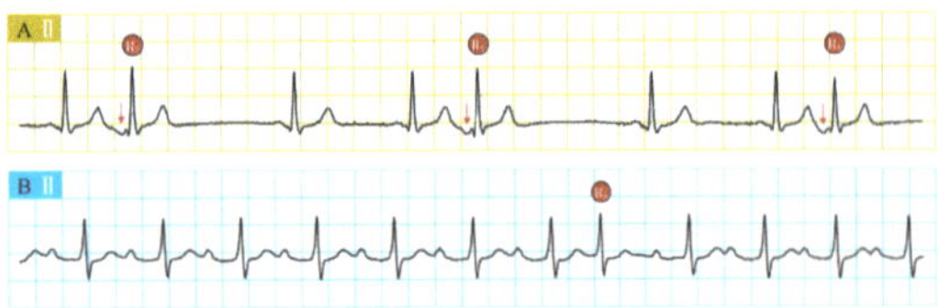

Premature junctional contraction

There may be no retrograde P wave, or there may be retrograde P wave, which appears before, hidden in or after QRS wave

Tx:

Sinus Arrythmia:

Sx: Usually asymptomatic

PE:

Dx: EKG

Tx:

Atrial Fibrillation: **Irregularly irregular**

Sx: Palpitations, hypotension, irregular pulse rate

PE:

Dx:

Tx:

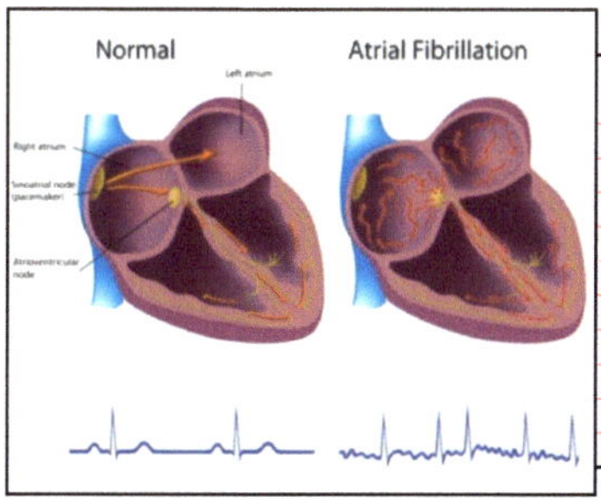

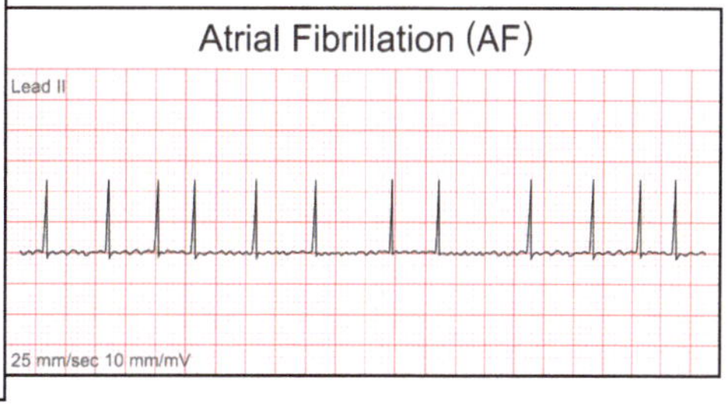

Atrial Flutter:

Sx:

PE:

Dx: EKG sawtooth pattern

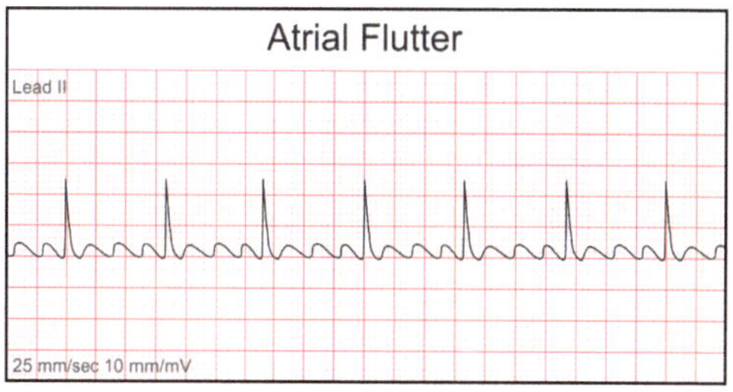

Tx:

Supraventricular Tachycardia:

Sx: Palpitations, abrupt onset & termination

PE:

Dx:

Tx:

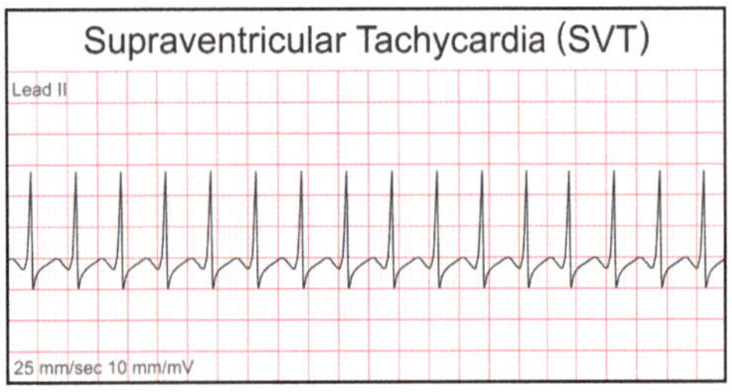

Wolf Parkinson White: Bundle of Kent

Draw the rhythm

Sx:

PE:

Dx: EKG = delta waves

Tx:

Long QT:

Draw the rhythm

Sx:

PE:

Dx: EKG = long QT interval

Tx:

Ventricular Tachycardia:

Most common cause:

Sx:

PE:

Dx: 3 or more PVCs, HR > 120

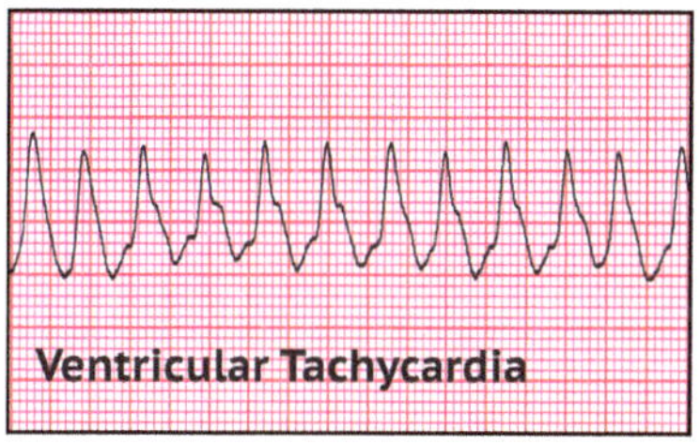

Tx:

Torsades de Pointes:

Most common cause: Hypomagnesaemia

Sx:

PE:

Dx: EKG = twisting around base

Tx:

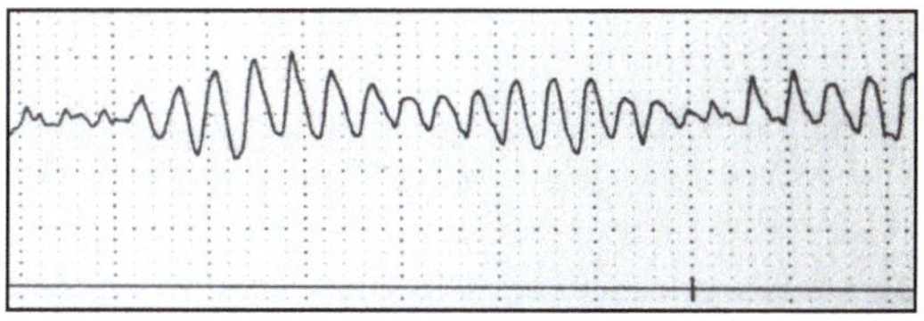

Ventricular Fibrillation: **Quivering of ventricles**

Sx:

PE:

Dx: EKG

Tx:

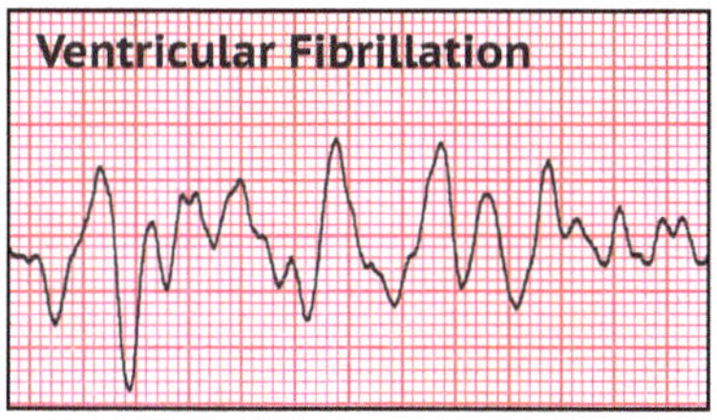

Vascular Disorders

Chronic Peripheral Arterial Disease:

Sx: Claudication, weak pedal pulses, leg hair stops growing, lower leg ulcers

PE:

Dx: US, arteriography, ankle brachial index < 0.90

______________________________ **Tx:**

____

____

Acute Peripheral Arterial Disease: Limb occlusion

Sx: 6 Ps (pain, pallor, poikilothermia, pulselessness, paresthesia, and paralysis)

PE:

Dx:

______________________________ **Tx:**

____

____

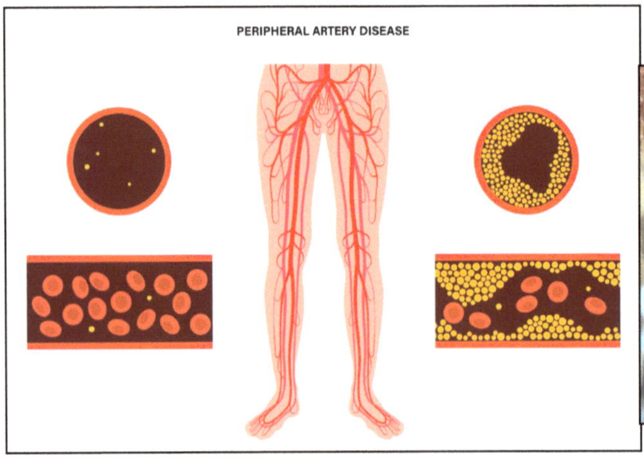

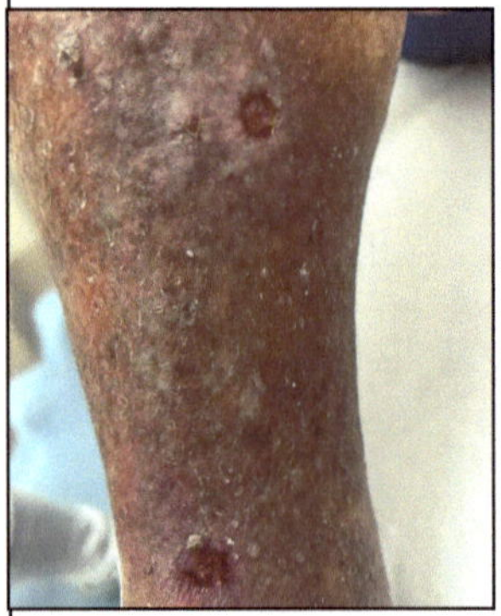

Abdominal Aortic Aneurysm:

Risk Factors: Age, smoking

Sx:

PE: Pulsatile mass

Dx:

Tx:

Thoracic Aortic Aneurysm:

Sx: Dyspnea, dysphagia, cough, hoarseness

PE:

Dx: Angiography

Tx:

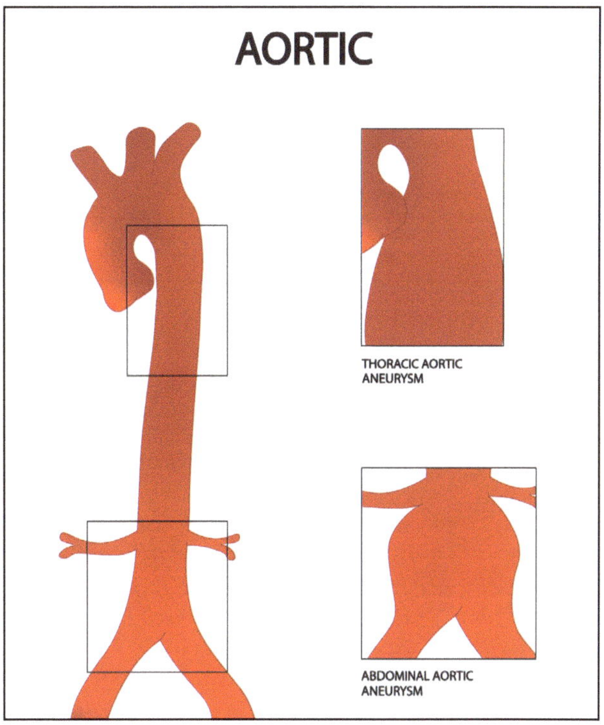

Aortic Dissection:

Sx: Tear of intima, ripping chest pain, decreased asymmetric pulses

Type A = proximal

Type B = distal

PE:

Dx: CT, MRA, transesophageal echocardiogram, Chest X-ray with widening of mediastinum

Tx:

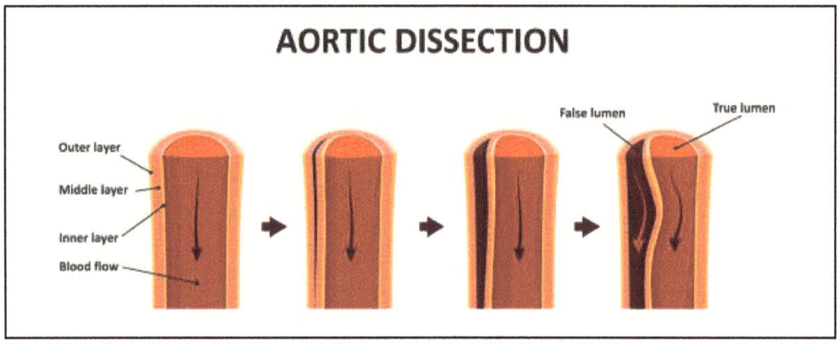

Arteriovenous Malformation (AVM): Brain & peripheral

Sx:

PE:

Dx: Vascular imaging (angiography)

Tx:

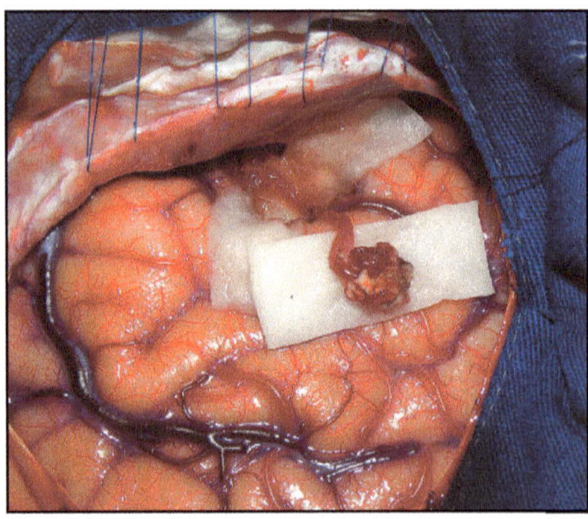

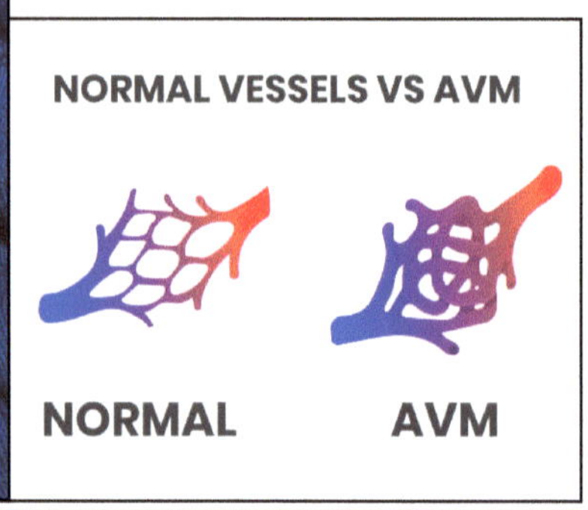

Giant Cell (Temporal) Arteritis: Associated with polymyalgia rheumatica

Sx: Headache, jaw claudication, tender, vision loss

PE:

Dx: ESR > 100, temporal artery biopsy

Tx:

Deep Vein Thrombosis (DVT):

Virchow's Triad
Stasis, hypercoagulable, trauma

Sx: Pain, erythema

PE: Positive Homan's sign

Dx:

Tx:

Superficial Vein Thrombophlebitis (Phlebitis): Inflammation leading to clot

Sx:

PE: Palpable cord

Dx: Venous US

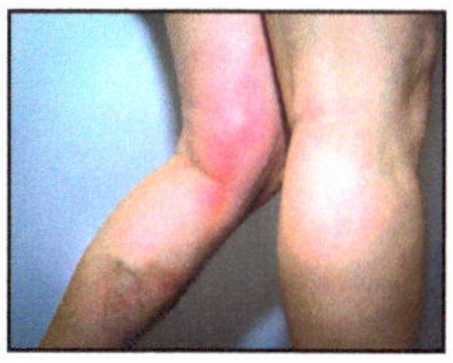

Tx:

Acute Mesenteric Ischemia:

Sx: Sudden abdominal pain

PE:

Dx: CTA, MRA, or CT without contrast

Tx:

Chronic Mesenteric Ischemia:

Sx: Postprandial pain

PE:

Dx: CTA, MRA, or duplex US

Tx:

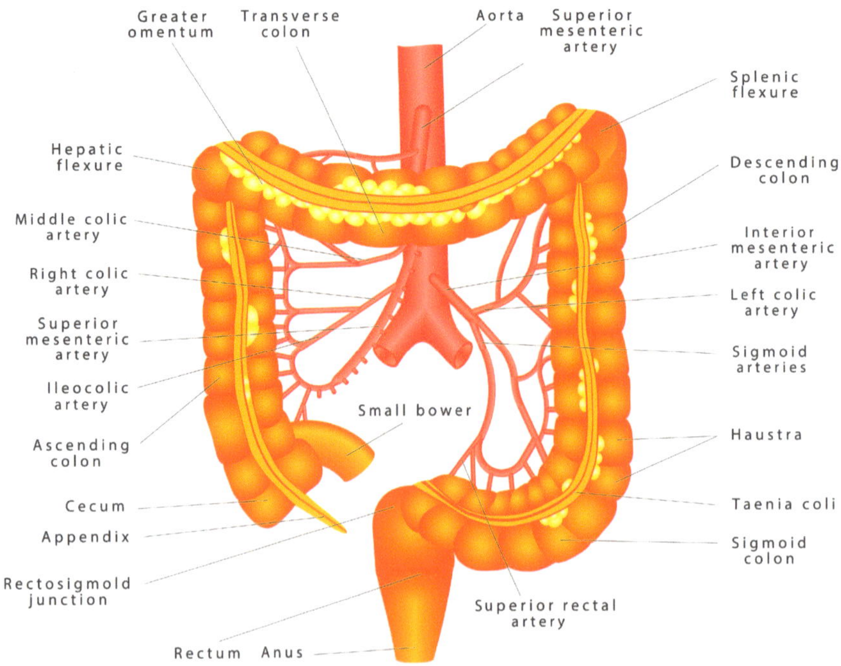

BLOOD SUPPLY TO THE COLON

Buerger's Disease (Thromboangiitis Obliterans): Inflammatory vasculitis + vaso-occlusion (young smoker)

Sx: Claudication, gangrene

PE:

Dx:

Tx:

Raynaud's: Arteriole vasospasm

Sx: White, blue, red fingers

PE:

Dx:

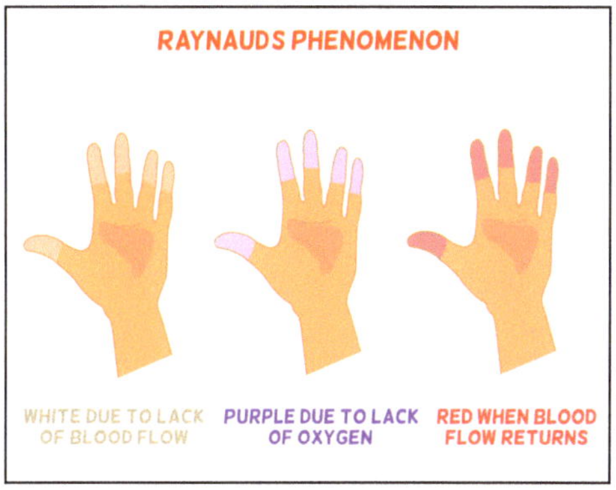

Tx:

Varicose Veins: Great saphenous vein most commonly affected

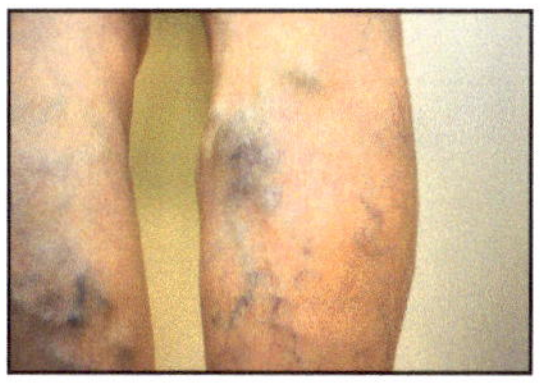

Sx: Dilated, tortuous veins, pain with standing, edema

PE:

Dx:

Tx:

Venous Insufficiency: Stasis dermatitis

Sx: Red/brown pigmented ulcers @ medial malleolus

PE:

Dx: US to rule out DVT

____

____

____

Tx:

Carotid Occlusive Disease: Atherosclerotic plaques

Sx: Bruit, TIA

PE:

Dx: US, angiography

____

____

____

Tx:

Hypertension, Cardiomyopathy, Heart Failure

Essential Hypertension:

Sx: Often asymptomatic

PE: Normal: **Elevated:**

Stage 1: **Stage 2:**

Dx: Labs:

UA:

EKG:

Tx:

JNC Treatment Targets:

ASCVD Risk Calculator:

Secondary Hypertension: Can be due to kidney disease, endocrine disorders, cardiac issues, sleep apnea, obesity, medications, etc.

Risk Factors:

Sx:

PE: Elevated BP

Dx:

Tx:

Hypertensive Urgency: > 180/120 without end-organ damage

Sx: May be asymptomatic, often will have headache

PE:

Dx:

Tx:

Hypertensive Emergency: > 180/120 with end-organ damage

Sx: Neurological symptoms, nausea, vomiting

PE: Fundoscopic changes

Dx:

Tx:

Malignant Hypertension (Hypertensive Crisis): Rapid elevation in BP with poor prognosis

Sx:

PE: Papilledema, encephalopathy, nephropathy, & A/V nicking

Dx:

Tx:

Hypotension

Cardiogenic Shock:

Sx: Hypotension, tachycardia, tachypnea

PE:

Dx:

Tx:

Orthostatic Hypotension:

Sx: Can be asymptomatic or experience dizziness, lightheadedness, and/or syncope

PE:

Dx:

Tx:

Vasovagal Syncope: Most common cause of syncope

Sx: Hypotension, bradycardia, syncope with vagal maneuvers

PE:

Dx:

Tx:

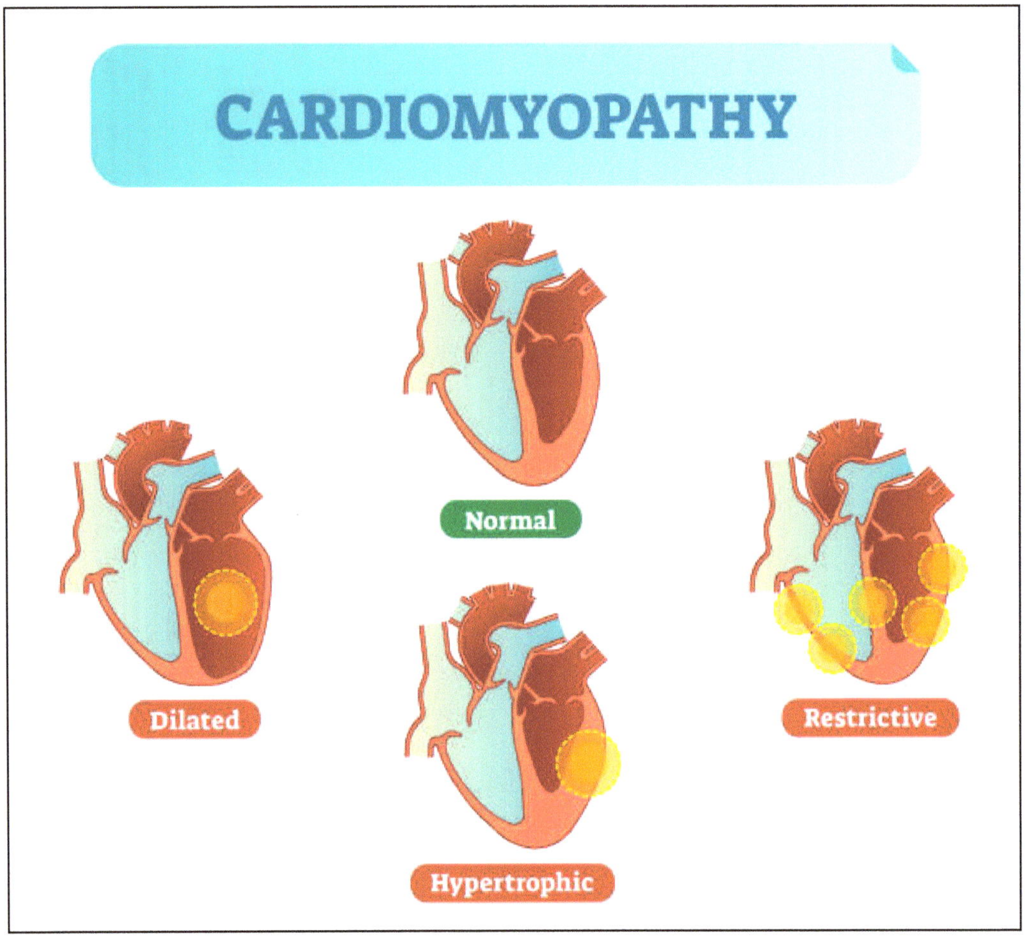
CARDIOMYOPATHY
Normal
Dilated
Restrictive
Hypertrophic

Dilated Cardiomyopathy: Enlargement primarily of left ventricle, with decreased wall thickness

All 4 chambers may be dilated in late stages

Causes: CAD, viral, EtOH, cocaine, OSA

Sx:

PE: S3, rales, JVD

Dx: Low ejection fraction < 50%

Tx:

Hypertrophic Cardiomyopathy: Thick LV (commonly septum), impaired outflow, sudden death in athlete

Sx: SOB, palpitations, syncope, family history

Murmur:

Dx:

Tx:

Restrictive Cardiomyopathy: Diastole, filling problem, normal ejection fraction

Associated with sarcoid and amyloidosis

Sx:

PE: S4, Kussmaul

Dx: Biopsy

Tx:

Left Ventricular Systolic Heart Failure: (Pumping issue)

Sx: Tachycardia, narrow pulse pressure, diaphoresis, vasoconstriction

PE:

Dx: Ejection fraction < 40%, BNP > 400

Tx:

Left Ventricular Diastolic Heart Failure: (Filling issue)

Sx: Heart failure symptoms

PE:

Dx: Normal ejection fraction

Tx:

Right Heart Failure: Blood backups into the body

Sx: Edema, JVD, ascites

PE:

Dx:

Tx:

Congenital Heart Defects

Atrial Septal Defect:

Sx:

Murmur:

Dx: EKG = RBBB

____

____

____

Tx:

Ventricular Septal Defect:

Sx:

Murmur:

Dx: EKG, Chest X-ray, transthoracic echocardiogram

____

____

____

Tx:

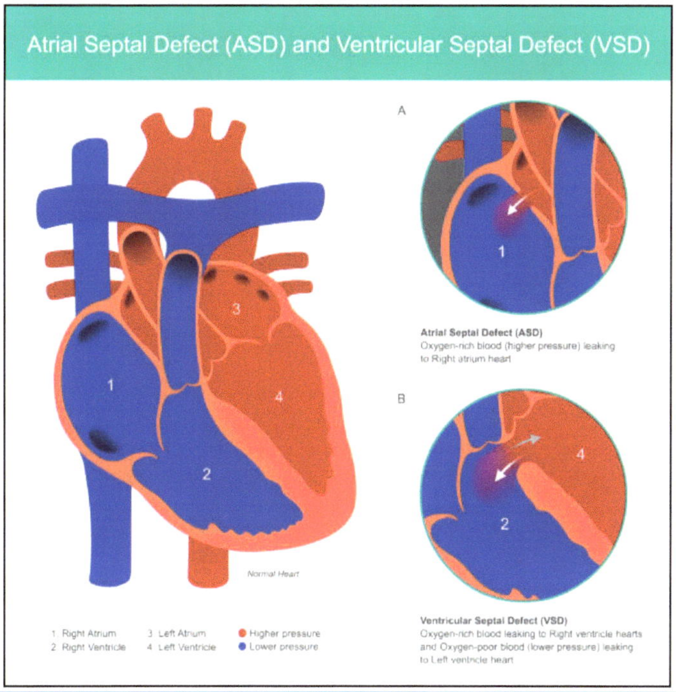

Coarctation of Aorta: Narrowing of aorta

Sx:

PE: Asymmetric BP/pulse

Dx: Rib notching on Chest X-ray

Tx:

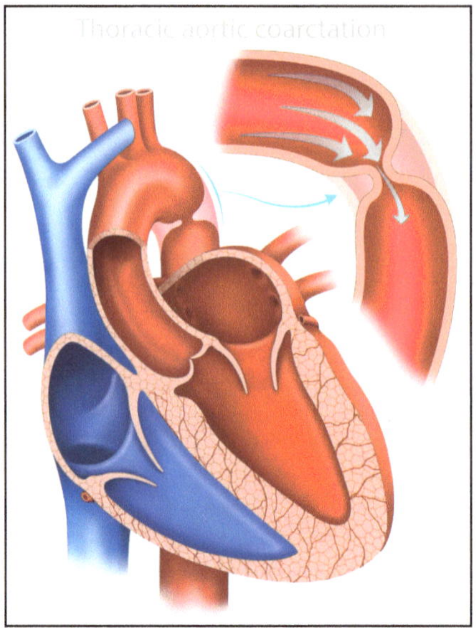

Patent Ductus Arteriosus: Should close in 1st week of life, failure to thrive

Sx: Bounding arterial pulse, cyanosis

Murmur:

Dx: EKG, echocardiogram

Tx:

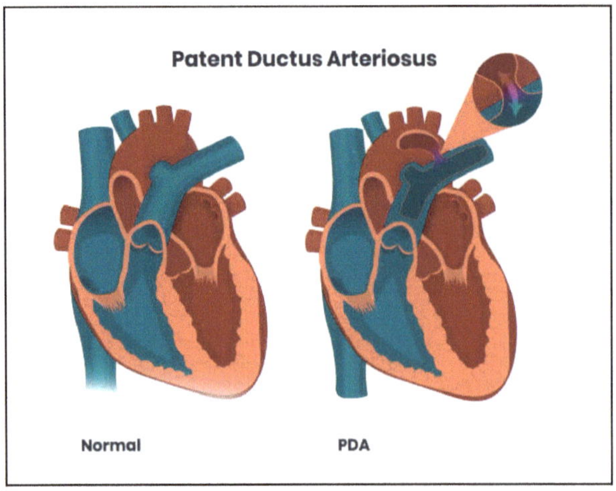

Tetralogy of Fallot: Left to right shunting

Sx: TET spells

Murmur:

Dx: Chest X-ray = boot shaped heart, left to right shunting

Tx:

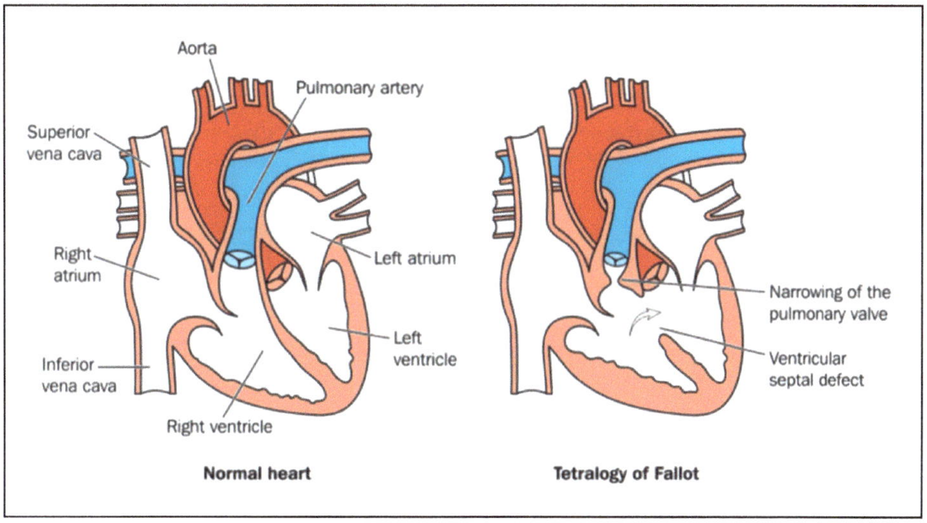

Atrial Myxoma: Benign, rare cardiac tumor

Sx:

PE:

Dx: Echocardiogram, EKG, Chest X-ray

Tx:

Lipid Disorders

Hypercholesterolemia: Elevated total cholesterol, LDL, triglycerides - can be hereditary

Sx: Asymptomatic, xanthelasma

PE:

Dx: Hereditary = genetic testing

Labs = total cholesterol > 200, LDL > 100-130, HDL < 45

Tx:

Hypertriglyceridemia:

Sx:

PE:

Dx: Labs = triglycerides > 150

Tx:

Hypertension Medications

Alpha Blocker

Alpha 1

Indications:

SE:

Alpha 2 agonist

Indications:

SE:

Beta Blockers "olol"

Beta 1- (crosses blood brain barrier)

Indications:

SE:

Black Box Warning

ACE Inhibitors "pril"

Indications:

SE:

ARB "sartan" (young, white)

Indications:

SE:

Renin Inhibitor

Indications:

SE:

Black Box Warning

Calcium Channel Blocker: **First line for black people & elderly - works on smooth muscle/visceral organs**

Non-Dihydropyridines:

Indications:

SE:

Dihydropyridines: "dipines"

Indications:

SE:

Black Box Warning

Direct Acting Vasodilators

Indications:

SE:

Nitrates

Indications:

SE:

Diuretic

Early Distal Tubule	Loop of Henley	Far Distal Tubule
Thiazides: K+ wasting	Loops:	K-sparing:
Indications:	Indications:	Indications:
SE:	SE:	SE:

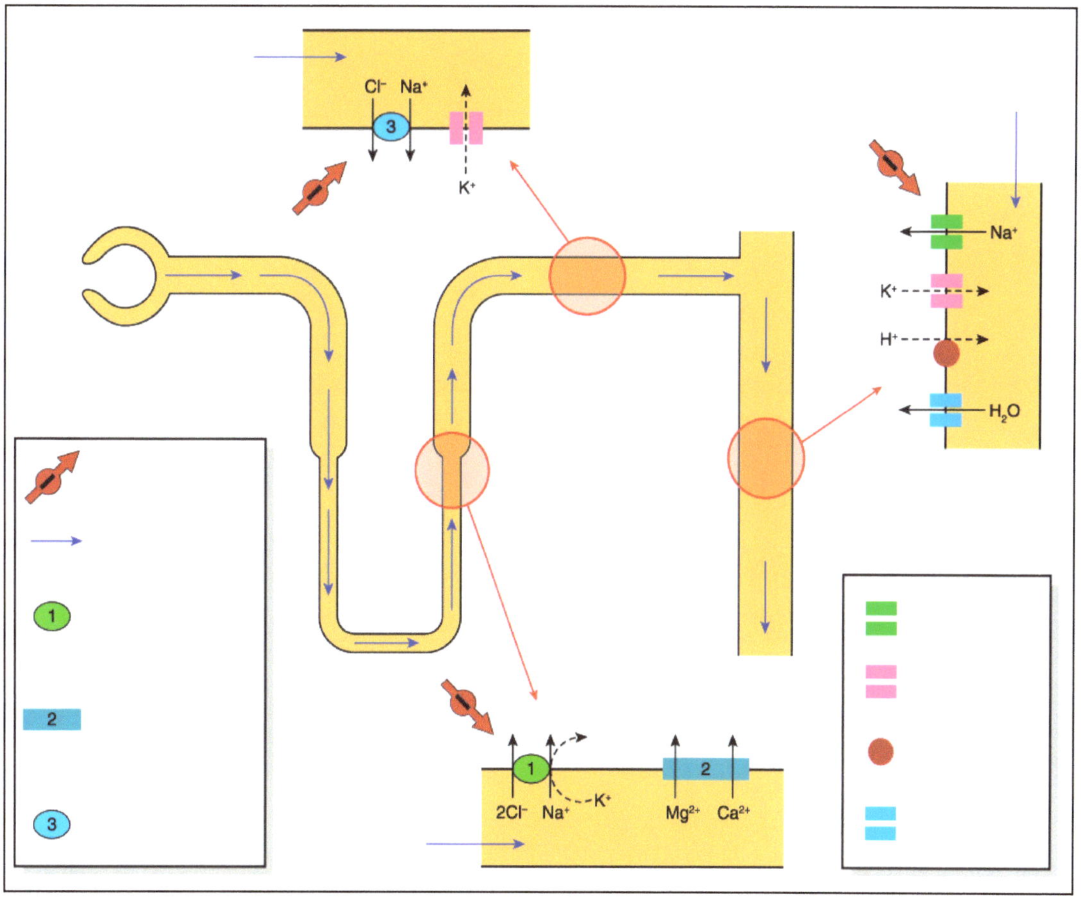

Anticoagulation

Vitamin K (Reversal) - PT/INR

Indications:

SE:

Heparins - PT

Indications:

SE:

Heparin Induced Thrombocytopenia (HIT) – PE or DVT

Direct Oral Anticoagulants - DOAC (also called NOAC - Novel Oral Anticoagulants)

Indications:

SE:

Anti-Platelets - Inhibits thrombus formation

TxA2 **P2Y12** **Aspirin** **Cox** **PDE III**

Indications:

SE:

Clotting Cascade

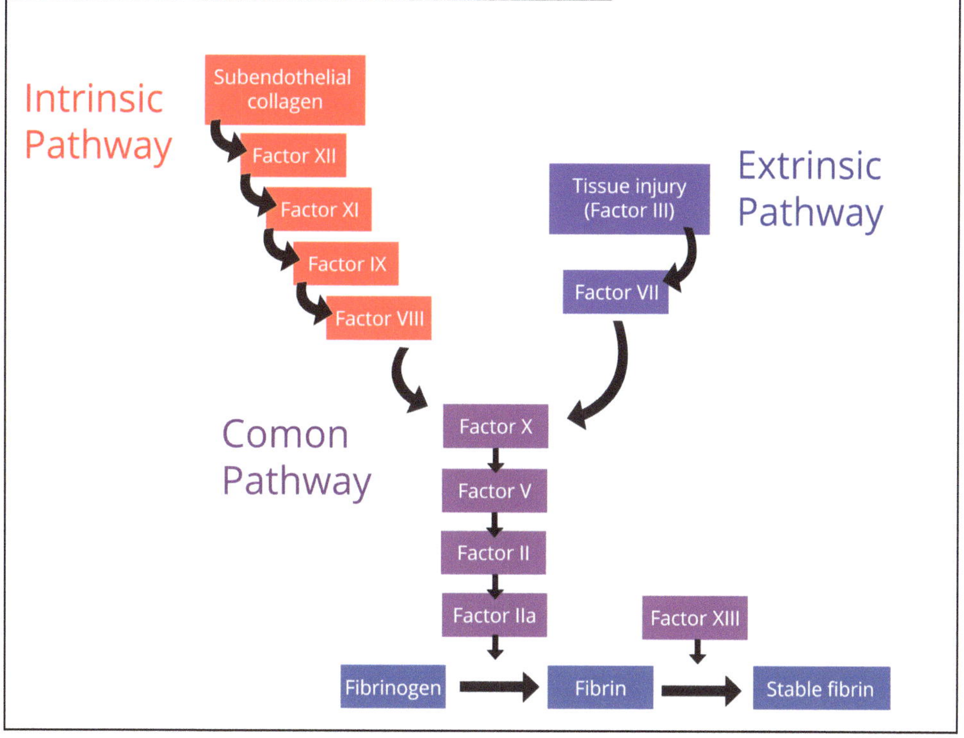

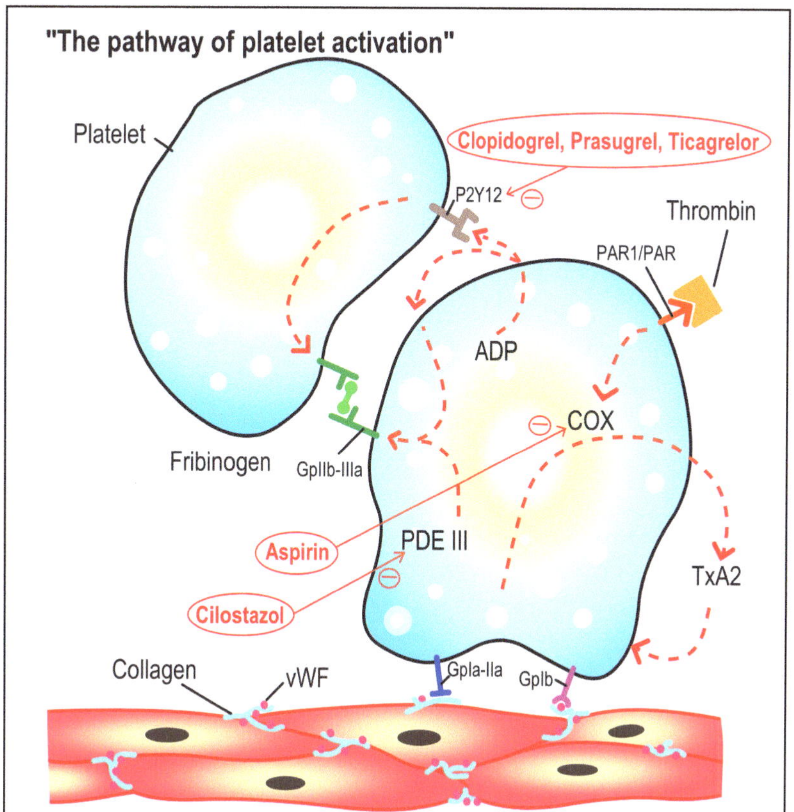

Hypercholesterolemia Medications

Statins: Reduce cholesterol synthesis

SE:

Indications:

PCSK9 Inhibitors

SE:

Indications:

Bile Acid Sequestrants:

SE:

Indications:

Niacin:

SE:

Indications:

Ezetimibe:

SE:

Indications:

Fibrates: Lower triglycerides

SE:

Indications:

Medications

____________________: **MOA =** ____

Indication(s) = ____

Side Effects = ____

Types/ Examples = ____

____________________: **MOA =** ____

Indication(s) = ____

Side Effects = ____

Types/ Examples = ____

____________________: **MOA =** ____

Indication(s) = ____

Side Effects = ____

Types/ Examples = ____

____________________: **MOA =** ____

Indication(s) = ____

Side Effects = ____

Types/ Examples = ____

____________________: **MOA =** ____

Indication(s) = ____

Side Effects = ____

Types/ Examples = ____

Medications

_______________: MOA = _______________

Indication(s) = _______________

Side Effects = _______________

Types/ Examples = _______________

_______________: MOA = _______________

Indication(s) = _______________

Side Effects = _______________

Types/ Examples = _______________

_______________: MOA = _______________

Indication(s) = _______________

Side Effects = _______________

Types/ Examples = _______________

_______________: MOA = _______________

Indication(s) = _______________

Side Effects = _______________

Types/ Examples = _______________

_______________: MOA = _______________

Indication(s) = _______________

Side Effects = _______________

Types/ Examples = _______________

Pulmonology

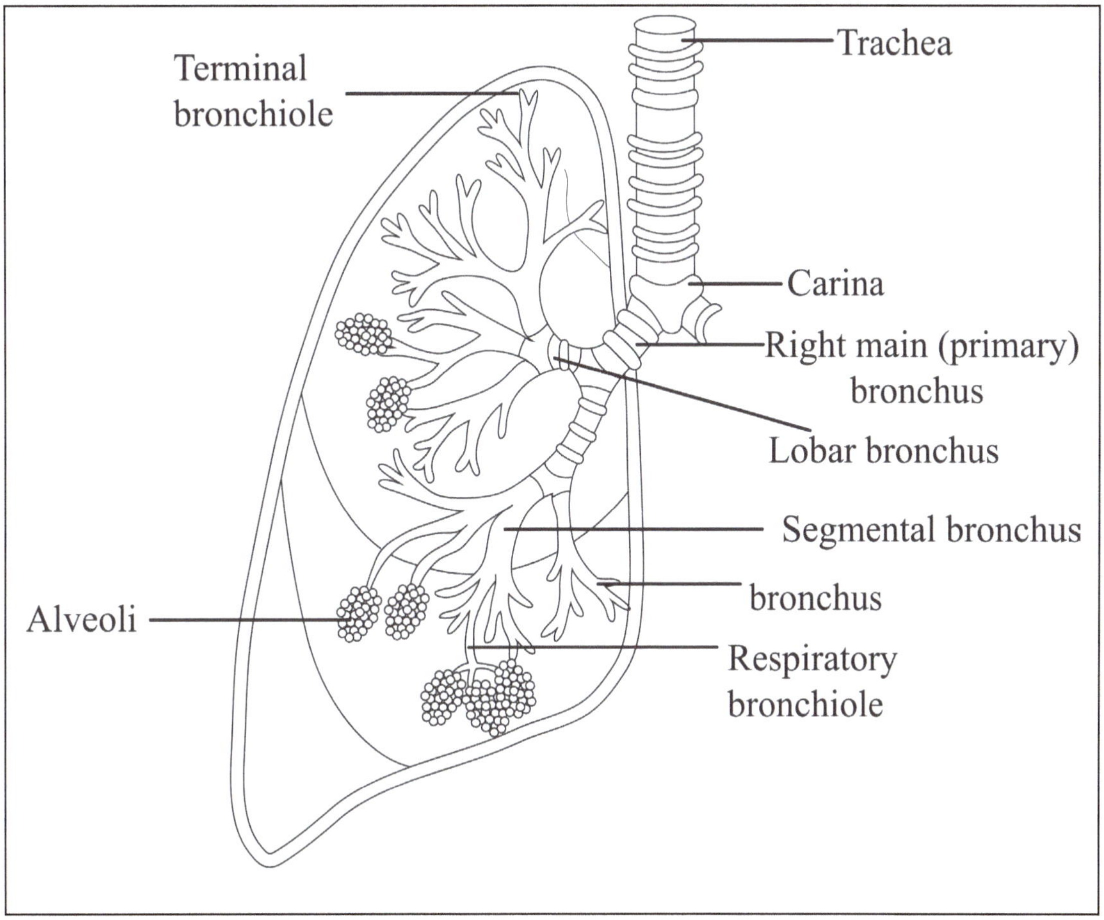

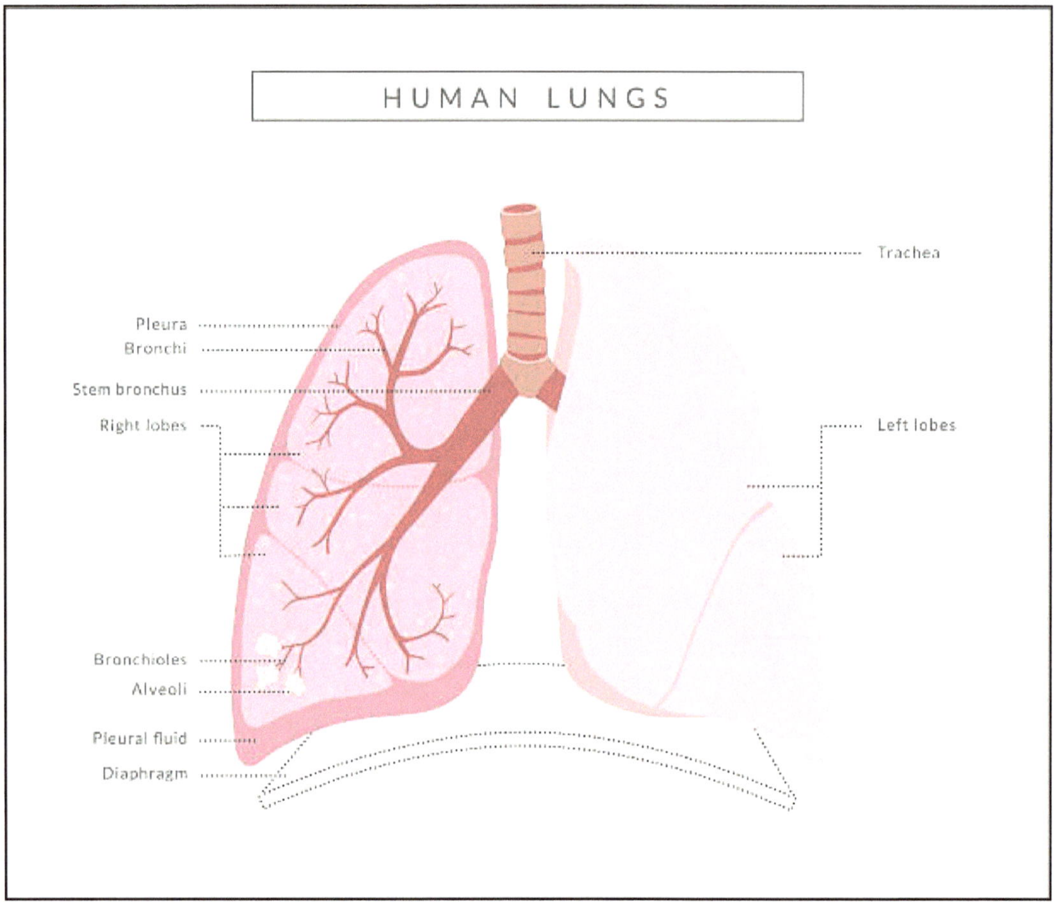
HUMAN LUNGS
Trachea
Pleura
Bronchi
Stem bronchus
Right lobes
Left lobes
Bronchioles
Alveoli
Pleural fluid
Diaphragm

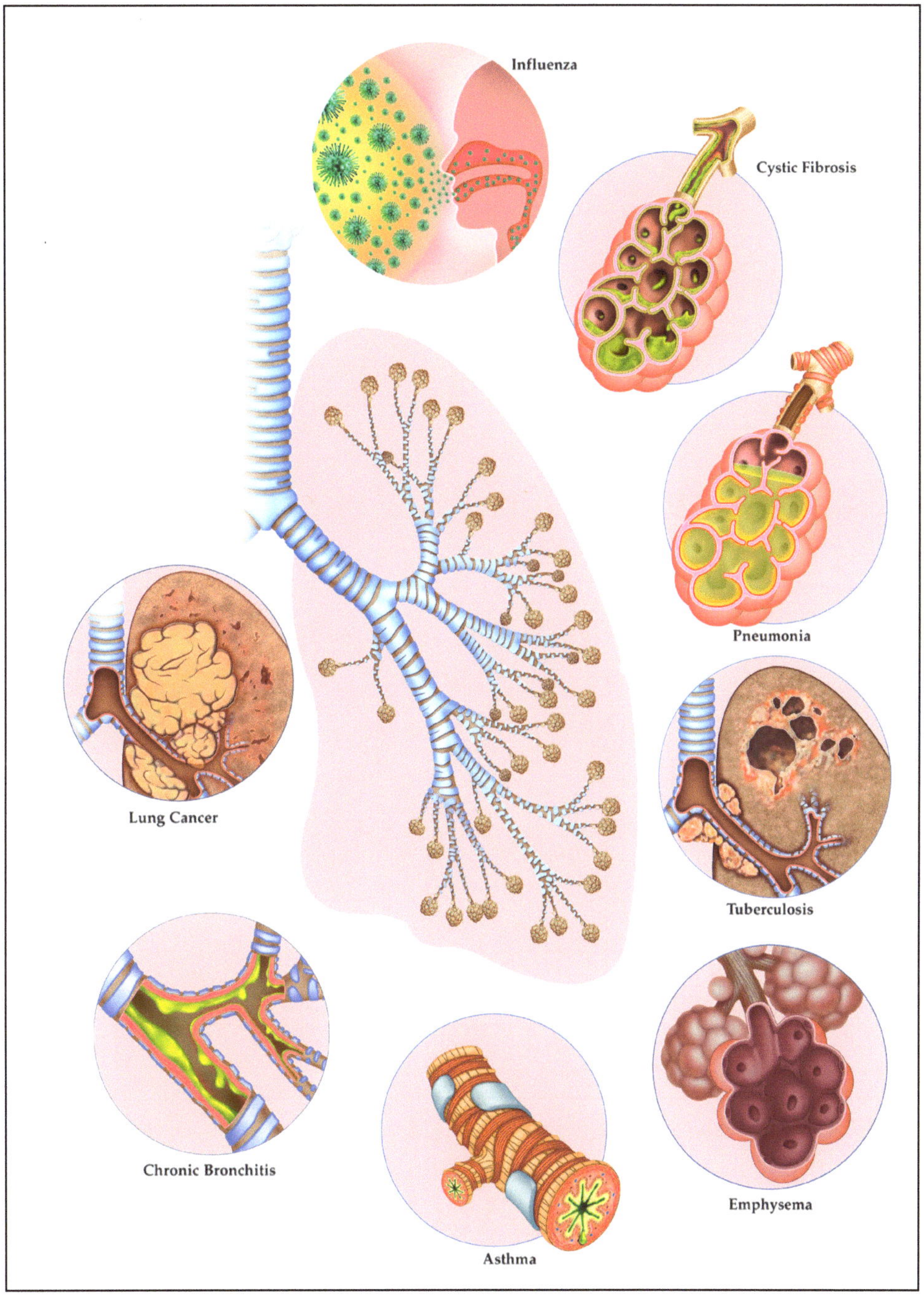
Influenza
Cystic Fibrosis
Pneumonia
Lung Cancer
Tuberculosis
Chronic Bronchitis
Asthma
Emphysema

Chronic Obstructive Pulmonary Disease:

Risk Factors:

1. Chronic Bronchitis 85%:

Sx: Chronic cough, productive sputum, dyspnea, prolonged expiration

PE: Rales, rhonchi, wheezing "Blue Bloaters"

2. Emphysema 15%:

Sx: Dyspnea, chronic cough (with or without sputum)

PE: Decreased breath sounds, barrel chest, hyperresonance, wheezing "Pink Puffer"

Dx:

Tx:

GOLD COPD Guidelines

Asthma:

Sx: Cough (more common at night), wheeze, shortness of breath

PE:

Dx: Low FEV1/FVC, normal DLCO

Tx:

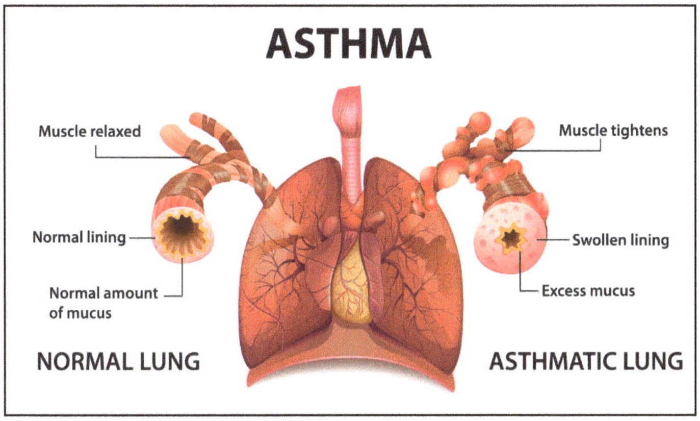

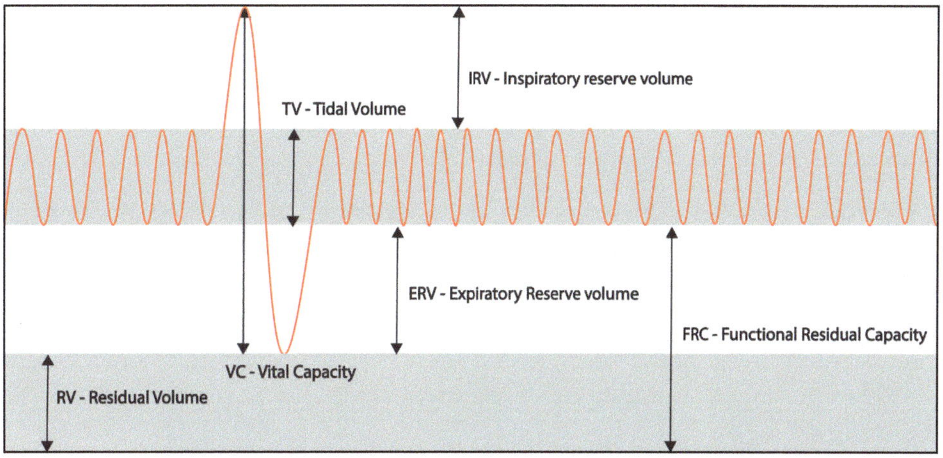

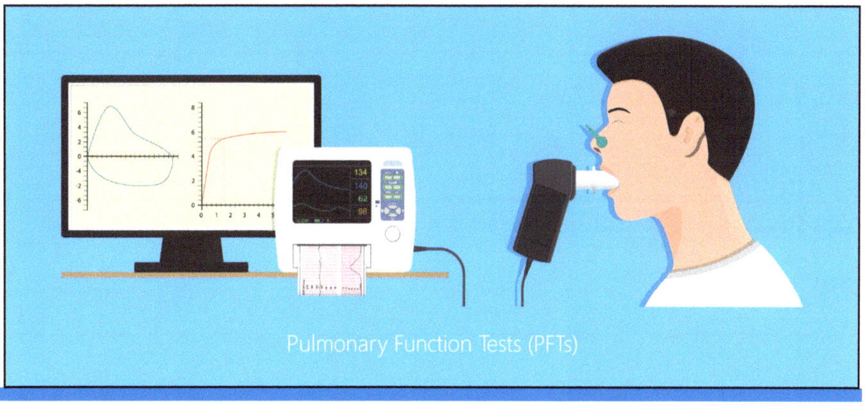

Obstructive Airway Medications

Beta 2 Agonist:
MOA = ____________________
Indication(s) = ____________________
Side Effects = ____________________
Types/ Examples = ____________________

____

____

Short Acting Beta Agonist (SABA):
MOA = ____________________
Indication(s) = ____________________
Side Effects = ____________________
Types/ Examples = ____________________

____

____

Long Acting Muscarinic Agonist (LAMA):
MOA = ____________________
Indication(s) = ____________________
Side Effects = ____________________
Types/ Examples = ____________________

____

____

Short Acting Muscarinic Agonist (SAMA):
MOA = ____________________
Indication(s) = ____________________
Side Effects = ____________________
Types/ Examples = ____________________

____

____

Inhaled Corticosteroids (ICS):
MOA = ____________________
Indication(s) = ____________________
Side Effects = ____________________
Types/ Examples = ____________________

____

____

Oral Glucocorticoid:

MOA = ______________________________

Indication(s) = ______________________________

Side Effects = ______________________________

Types/ Examples = ______________________________

____

____

Omalizumab:

MOA = ______________________________

Indication(s) = ______________________________

Side Effects = ______________________________

Types/ Examples = ______________________________

____

____

Mast Cell Stabilizers:

MOA = ______________________________

Indication(s) = ______________________________

Side Effects = ______________________________

Types/ Examples = ______________________________

____

____

Antileukotrienes:

MOA = ______________________________

Indication(s) = ______________________________

Side Effects = ______________________________

Types/ Examples = ______________________________

____

____

Antimuscarinics:

MOA = ______________________________

Indication(s) = ______________________________

Side Effects = ______________________________

Types/ Examples = ______________________________

____

____

Asthma management chart

Restrictive Pulmonary Disease

Restrictive pattern = normal or increased FEV 1/FVC, normal or decreased FVC, decreased lung volumes (VC, RV, FRC, TLC) decreased DLCO

Idiopathic Pulmonary Fibrosis: Progressive scarring of the lungs for unknown reasons

Sx:

PX: Fine, dry, bibasilar inspiratory crackles, clubbing

Dx:

Tx:

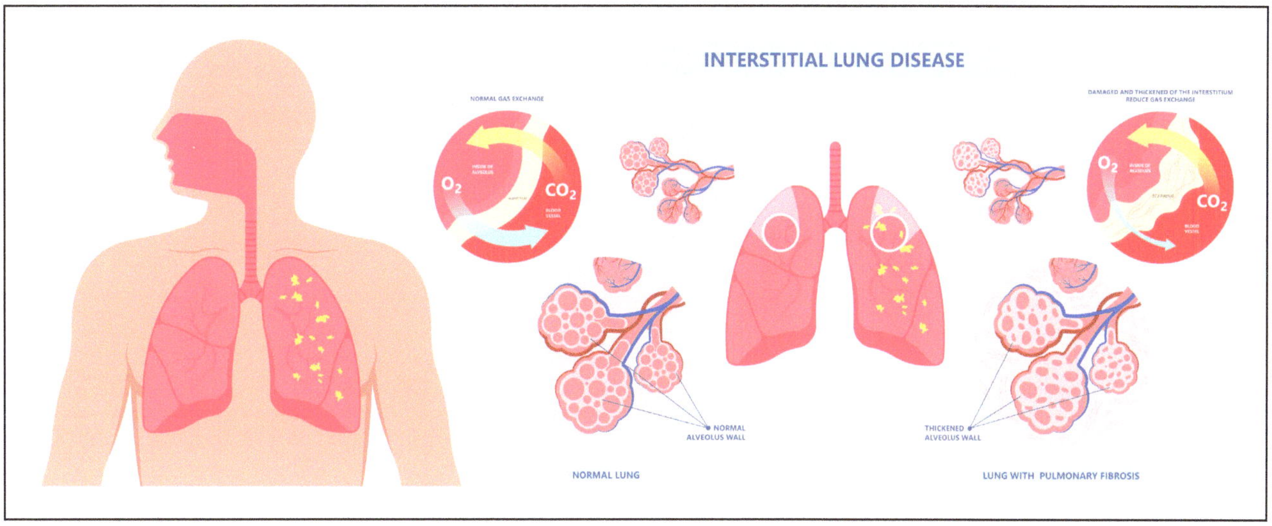

Pneumoconiosis

Asbestosis: **Diffuse, progressive pulmonary fibrosis**

Risk Factors:

Sx:

PE: Clubbing, bibasilar crackles

Dx:

______________________________ **Tx:**

____

____

Silicosis: **Inhalation of silicon dioxide (coal mining, granite, slate, quartz, sandblasting, stone mason)**

Sx: Chronic:

Acute:

PE: Crackles

Dx:

______________________________ **Tx:**

____

____

Berylliosis: **Granulomatous pulmonary disease caused by beryllium exposure**

Risk Factors:

Sx: Dyspnea, cough, fever, weight loss

PE:

Dx:

______________________________ **Tx:**

____

____

Coal Worker's Pneumoconiosis (Black Lung): Inhalation of coal dust

Sx:

PX: Crackles

Dx:

Tx:

Sarcoidosis:

Risk Factors: Females, African Americans, Northern Europeans

Sx:

PE: Lupus perino (specific), erythema nodosum (most common)

Dx: Bronchoscopy = gold standard

Tx:

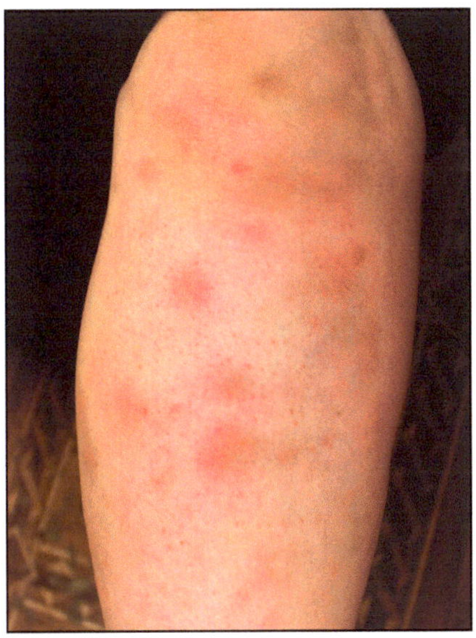

Erythema nodosum (most common)

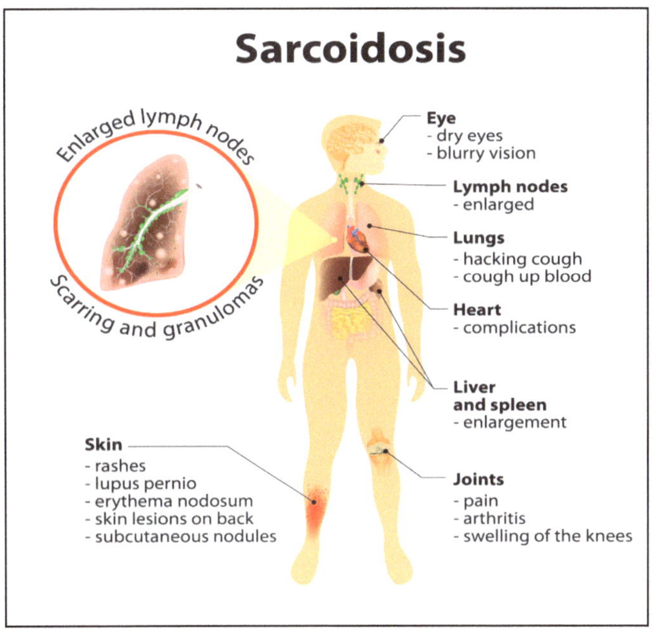

Infectious Pulmonary Disorders

Acute Bronchiolitis (RSV - Respiratory Syncytial Virus): Lower respiratory tract

Sx: Cough, fever, wheeze

PE:

Dx:

Tx:

Acute Bronchitis: Most common is viral

Sx: Cough 5-21 days, #1 cause of hemoptysis

PE:

Dx:

Tx:

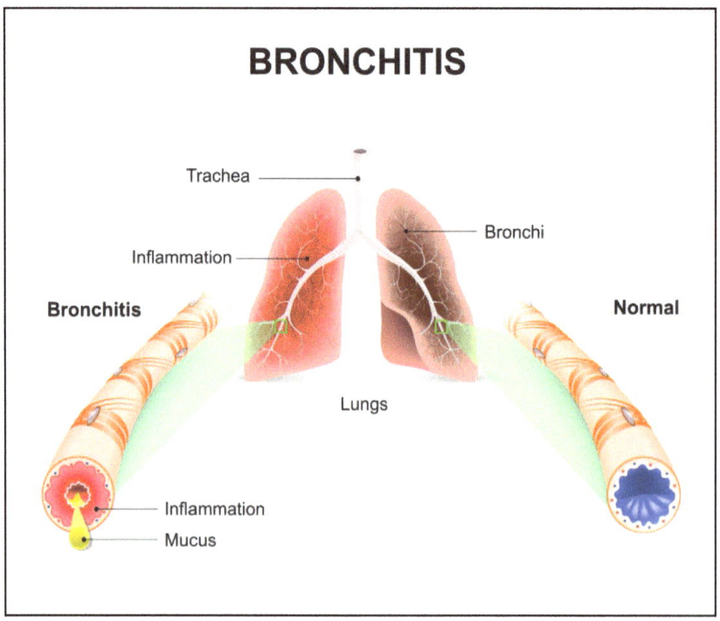

Pertussis "Whooping Cough": Bordetella pertussis - gram neg rod

3 stages:

Sx: Inspiratory stridor/whoop, emesis, fever

PE:

Dx: X-ray = perihilar infiltrates, atelectasis

______________________________ **Tx:**

____

____

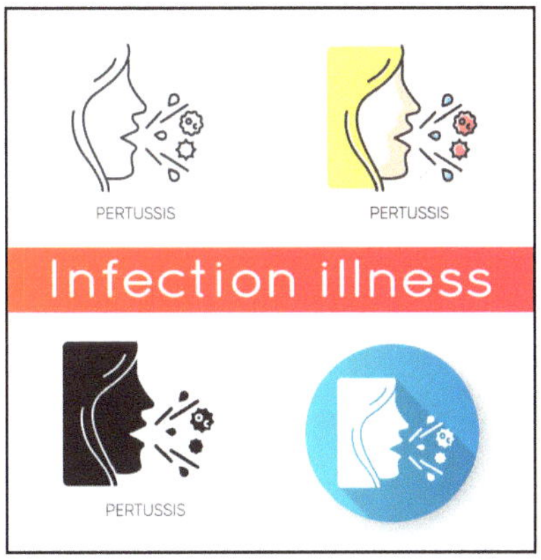

Vaccine:

Influenza A&B:

Sx: Fever, sore throat, cough, lymphadenopathy

PE:

Dx: Clinical, viral culture or rapid antigen test

______________________________ **Tx:**

____

____

Pneumonia:

Complications: Empyema, abscess

Sx: Productive cough, rales, decreased breath sounds, fever + WBC + infiltrate

PE:

Dx:

Tx:

Vaccine:

CURB 65

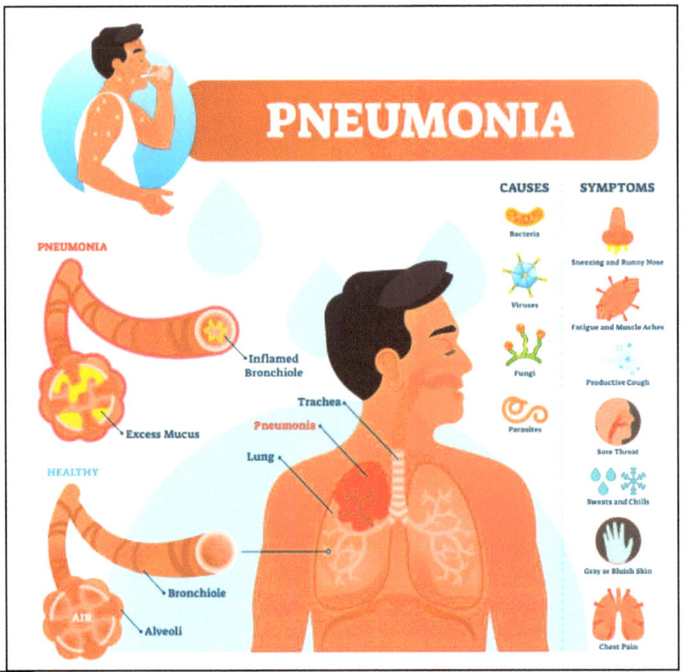

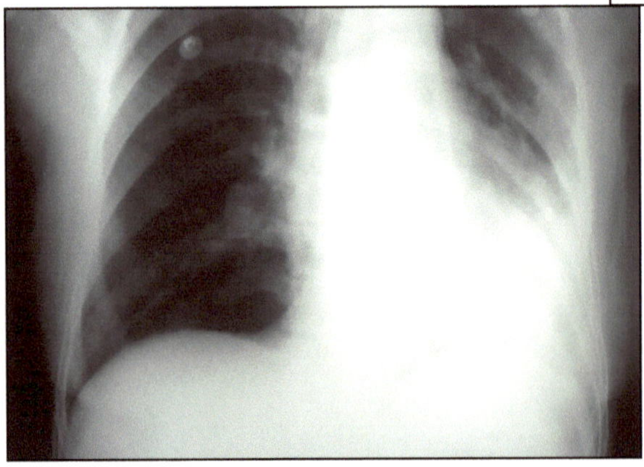

Bacterial Pneumonia

Pneumococcal Pneumonia: **Strep pneumoniae (gram-positive diplococci), community acquired pneumonia (CAP)**

Sx: Rust sputum

Dx:

Tx:

M. Catarrhalis: **COPD, elderly**

Sx: Systemic symptoms

Dx:

Tx:

Haemophilus Influenzae: **Gram negative - second most common cause of CAP**

Sx: Meningitis symptoms but no rash, HIB meningitis - seen in babies 6-24 months

Dx: Clinical, physical exam

Tx:

Atypical Pneumonia

Chlamydia Pneumoniae: **College kids, sore throat**

Sx: Cough, fever, rales

Dx:

Tx:

Legionella: **Air conditioning, water source**

Sx: Fever, headache, crackles/rhonchi, hyponatremia, diarrhea

Dx:

Tx:

Mycoplasma Pneumoniae: **"Walking pneumonia", school aged children, college students, military**

Sx:

Dx: X-ray = reticulonodular pattern, PCR, serology, cold agglutination

Tx:

Healthcare Acquired Pneumonia

Causes: IV wound care, hospitalized within 90 days, outpatient treatment in hospital (i.e., dialysis)

Pseudomonas: Green sputum

Sx:

Dx: X-ray = progressive infiltrates

Tx:

Other Pneumonia

Aspiration Pneumonia: Strep, staph, haemophilus influenzae, klebsiella, and anaerobes

Sx: Cough, dyspnea, fever, pleuritic chest pain

Dx:

Tx:

Viral Pneumonia: Inflammation of alveolar walls

Most Common Cause: Kids = RSV

Adults = influenza A & B, Covid

Sx: Afebrile

Dx: X-ray = diffuse infiltrates

Tx:

Tuberculosis: Mycobacterium

Sx: Hemoptysis, weight loss, night sweats, fever

PE:

Dx: Latent Dx:

Active Dx:

Tx:

TB testing:

PPD -

QuantiFERON Gold -

Chest X-ray -

Vaccine:

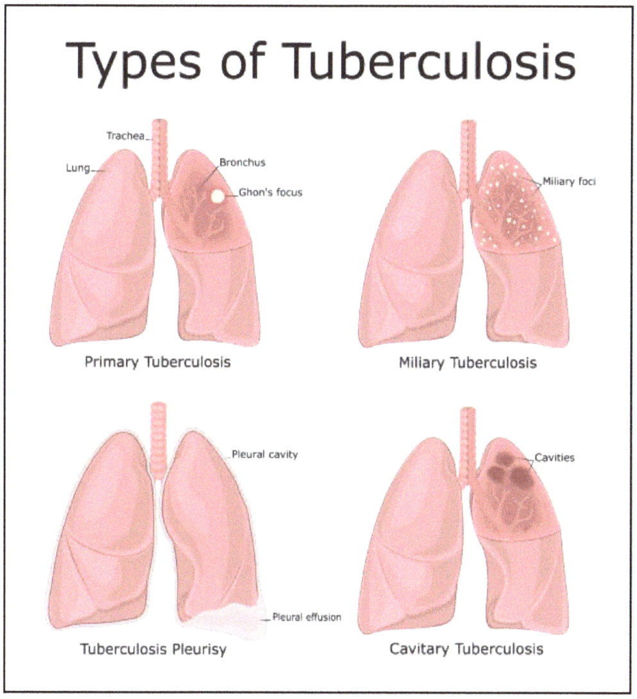

Bronchiectasis: **Permanent dilation and destruction of the airway, most common cause is cystic fibrosis**

Sx: Chronic cough, ***foul smelling sputum***, hemoptysis, clubbing, recurrent pneumonia

PE: Crackles, wheezing, rhonchi

Dx:

____

____

____

Tx:

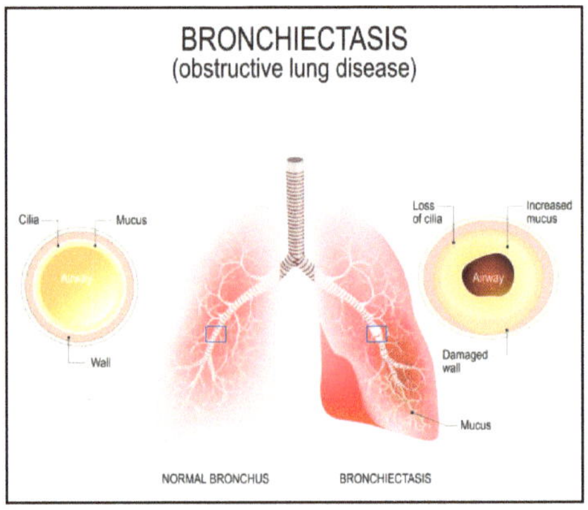

Lung Abscess: **Anaerobes, seen in alcoholics and those with epilepsy, most common in right lower lobe**

Sx: Cough, fever, chills, purulent sputum

PE:

Dx:

____

____

____

Tx:

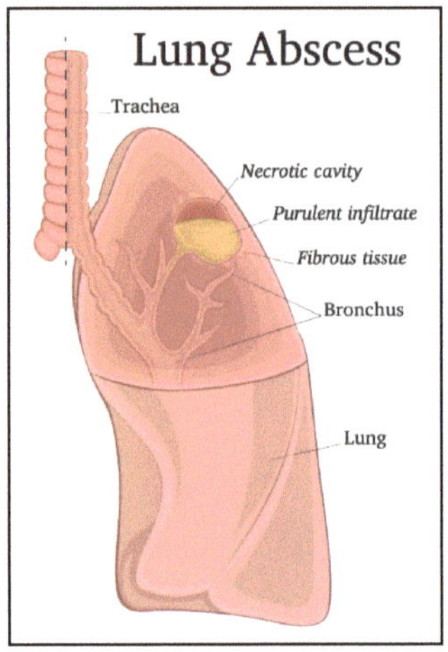

Empyema: **Purulent fluid in pleural space**

Sx: Persistent fever, recent pneumonia, constitutional symptoms

PE:

Dx:

____

____

____

Tx:

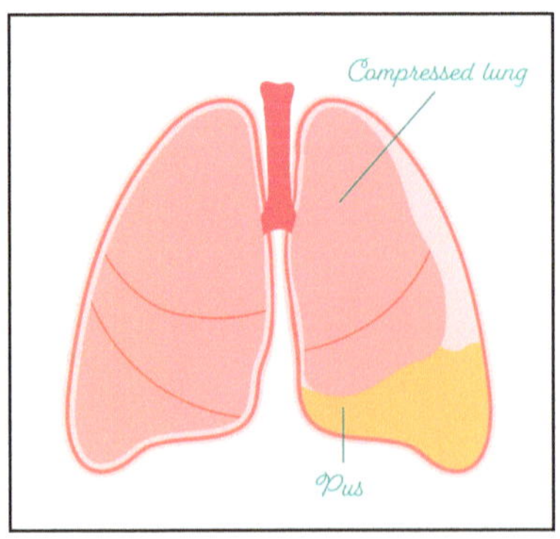

Pulmonic Nodules and Neoplasms

Small Cell Lung Cancer: Smoking #1 cause, aggressive

Sx: Hemoptysis, dyspnea, asymptomatic

PE:

Dx:

Tx:

Squamous Cell Lung Cancer: Non-small cell lung cancer, smoking

Sx: Hemoptysis, dyspnea, asymptomatic

PE:

Dx:

Tx:

Large Cell Lung Cancer:

Sx: Pleuritic pain, dyspnea, cough

PE:

Dx:

Tx:

Adenocarcinoma: Non-smokers

Sx: Pleuritic pain, dyspnea, cough

PE:

Dx:

Tx:

Pulmonary Nodules:

Sx: Can be asymptomatic, dyspnea, cough

PE: Round lesion that is > 3cm and surrounded by lung parenchyma

Dx:

Tx:

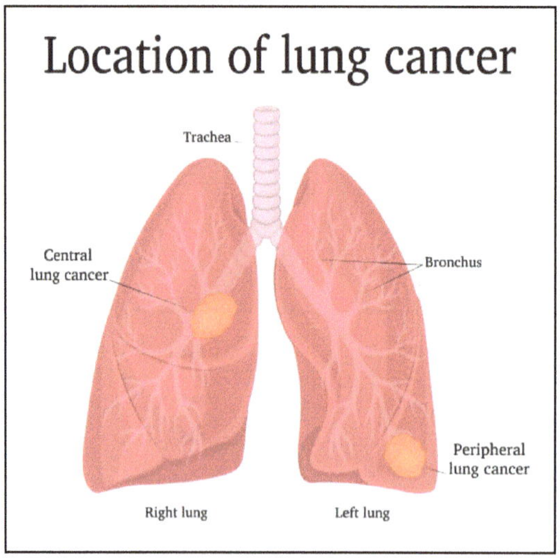

Pleural Diseases

Pleural Effusions: Fluid in pleural space

Sx:

PE:

Dx: X-ray, CT, thoracentesis

____

____

____

> **Pleural fluid analysis = Light's Criteria**
>
> **Gram stain/culture**
>
> **Transudate: More likely bilateral**
>
> **Exudate: More likely unilateral high protein, high LDH**

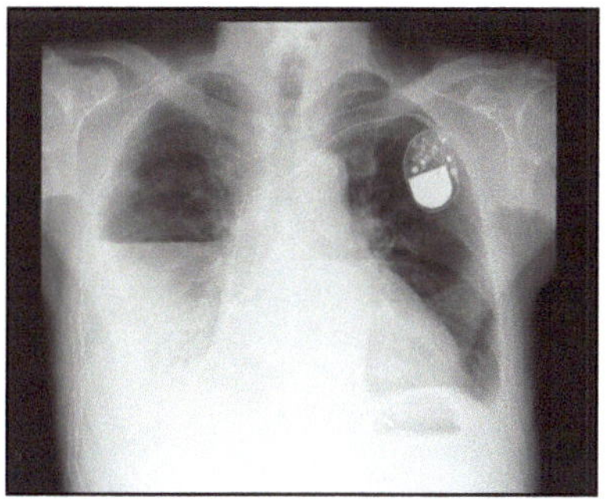

Tx: Depends on underlying cause

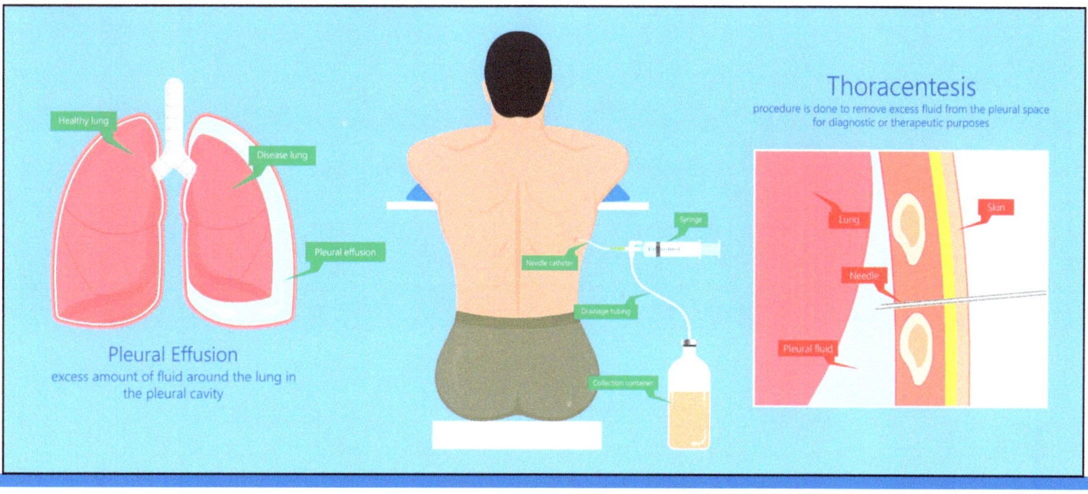

Pneumothorax: Air in pleural space

Sx: Acute chest pain, shortness of breath, decreased breath sounds, hyperresonance

Spontaneous=

Tension=

PE:

Dx:

____

____

____

Tx: Small:

Large:

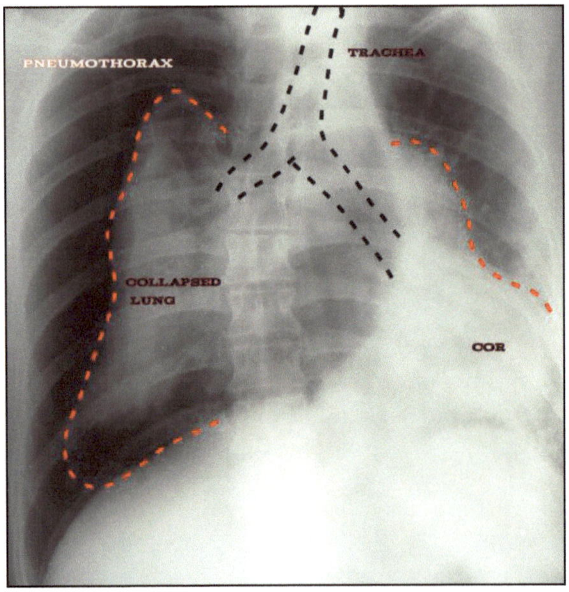

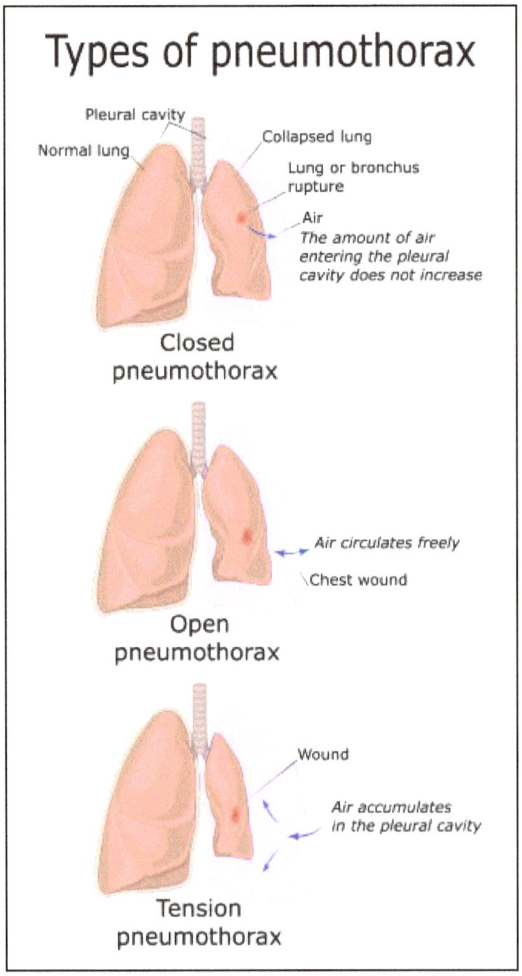

Pulmonary Circulation Disorders

Pulmonary Embolism:

Risk Factor:

Sx:

PE: Virchow's Triad:

Dx: CTA pulmonary angiogram = gold standard

X-ray:

EKG:

Tx:

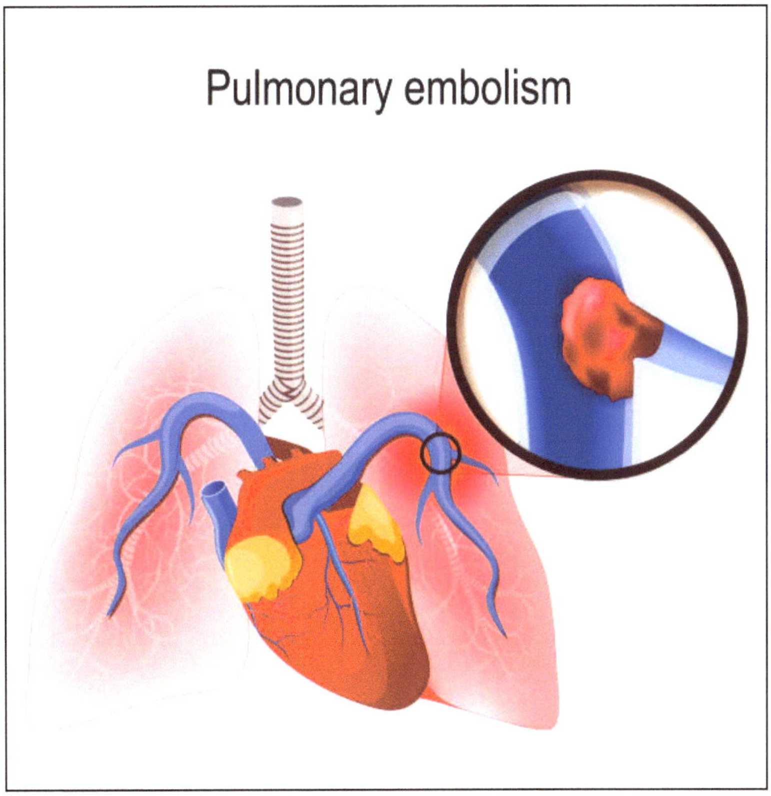

Pulmonary Hypertension: **Pulmonary artery pressure > 25 mmHg**

Sx: Right heart failure symptoms, shortness of breath, chest pain

PE:

Dx:

______________________________ **Tx:**

____

____

Primary/idiopathic: **Tx:**

Secondary: **Tx:**

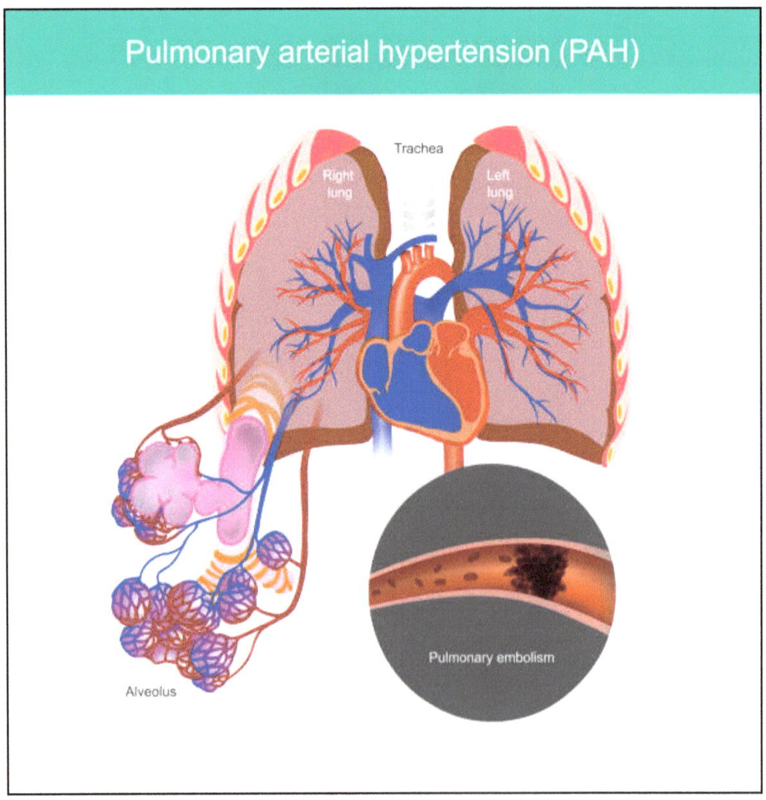

Sleep Apnea: Obstructive or central

Sx:

PE:

Dx: History, polysomnography

____

____

____

Tx:

Other Pulmonary Disorders

Acute Respiratory Distress Syndrome - *EMERGENCY*

Known as Respiratory Distress Syndrome or "Hyaline Membrane Disease" in preterm infants. Low Surfactant

Sx:

PE:

Dx: X-ray:

PaO2/FiO2: < 200

Wedge pressure:

Tx:

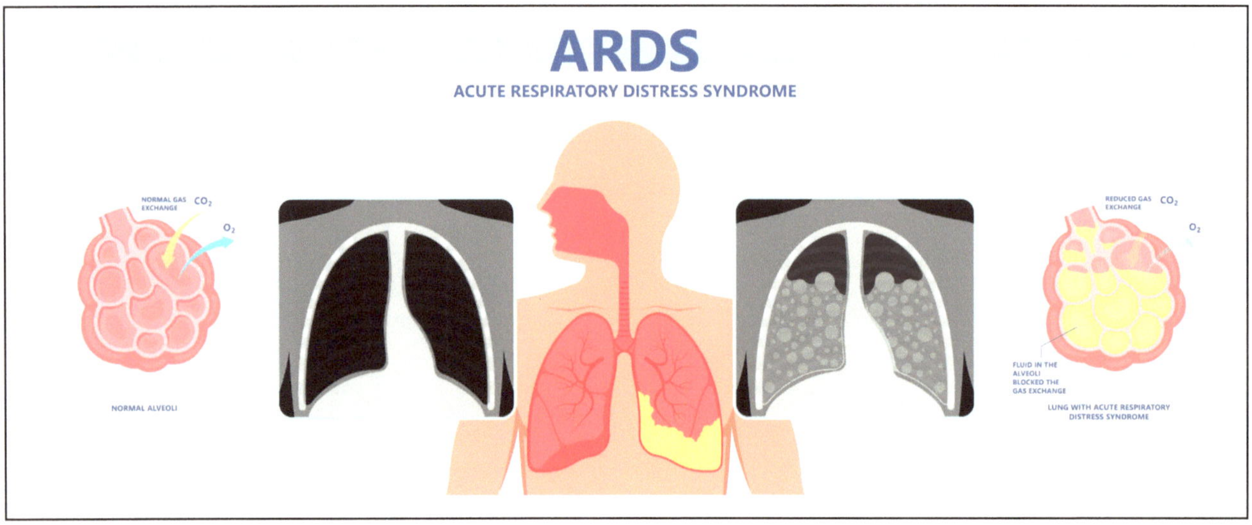

Samter's Triad:

Sx: Aspirin sensitivity + asthma + nasal polyps

PE:

Dx:

Tx:

Cystic Fibrosis: Autosomal recessive

Sx:

PE: Nasal polyps, pancreatic insufficiency

Dx: Sweat chloride test

Tx:

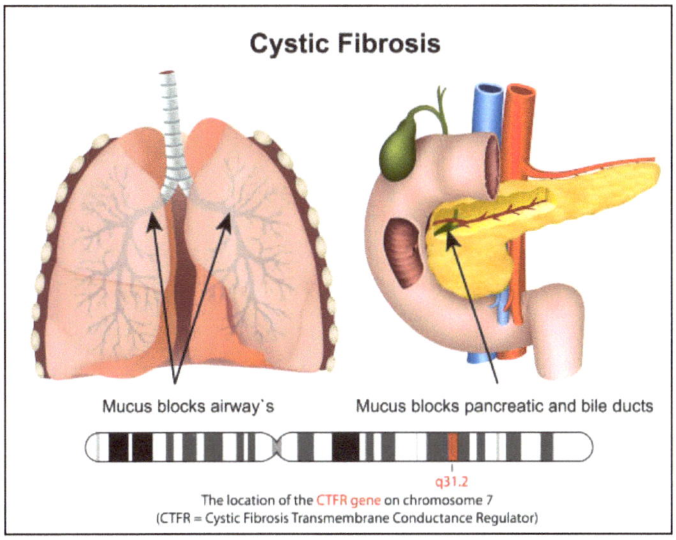

Foreign Body Aspiration: **Most common right side**

Sx: Stridor, cough, wheezing

PE:

Dx: X-ray can be normal, bronchoscopy

Tx:

Atelectasis: **Alveolar collapse, can be full or partial**

Sx: Trouble breathing, cough, chest pain

PE:

Dx: X-ray

Tx:

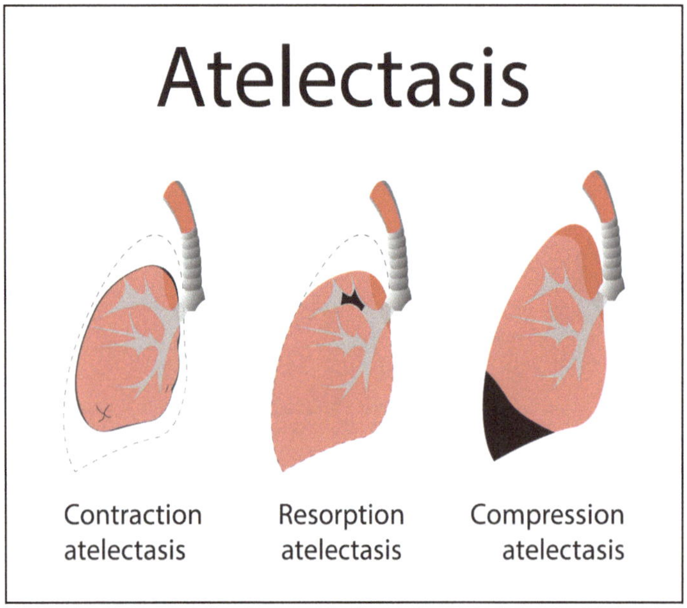

Obesity Hypoventilation Syndrome:

Sx: Daytime sleepiness, fatigue, impaired memory

PE: Obese body habitus

Dx:

___

___

___

Acute Epiglottitis: ***In EENT***

Croup (Parainfluenza): ***In EENT***

Medications

______________: MOA = ______________

Indication(s)=______________

Side Effects = ______________

Types/ Examples = ______________

____

____

______________: MOA = ______________

Indication(s)=______________

Side Effects = ______________

Types/ Examples = ______________

____

____

______________: MOA = ______________

Indication(s)=______________

Side Effects = ______________

Types/ Examples = ______________

____

____

______________: MOA = ______________

Indication(s)=______________

Side Effects = ______________

Types/ Examples = ______________

____

____

______________: MOA = ______________

Indication(s)=______________

Side Effects = ______________

Types/ Examples = ______________

____

____

Medications

___________________: MOA = ____

Indication(s)=____

Side Effects = ____

Types/ Examples = ____

____

____

___________________: MOA = ____

Indication(s)=____

Side Effects = ____

Types/ Examples = ____

____

____

___________________: MOA = ____

Indication(s)=____

Side Effects = ____

Types/ Examples = ____

____

____

___________________: MOA = ____

Indication(s)=____

Side Effects = ____

Types/ Examples = ____

____

____

___________________: MOA = ____

Indication(s)=____

Side Effects = ____

Types/ Examples = ____

____

____

Gastrointestinal Disorders

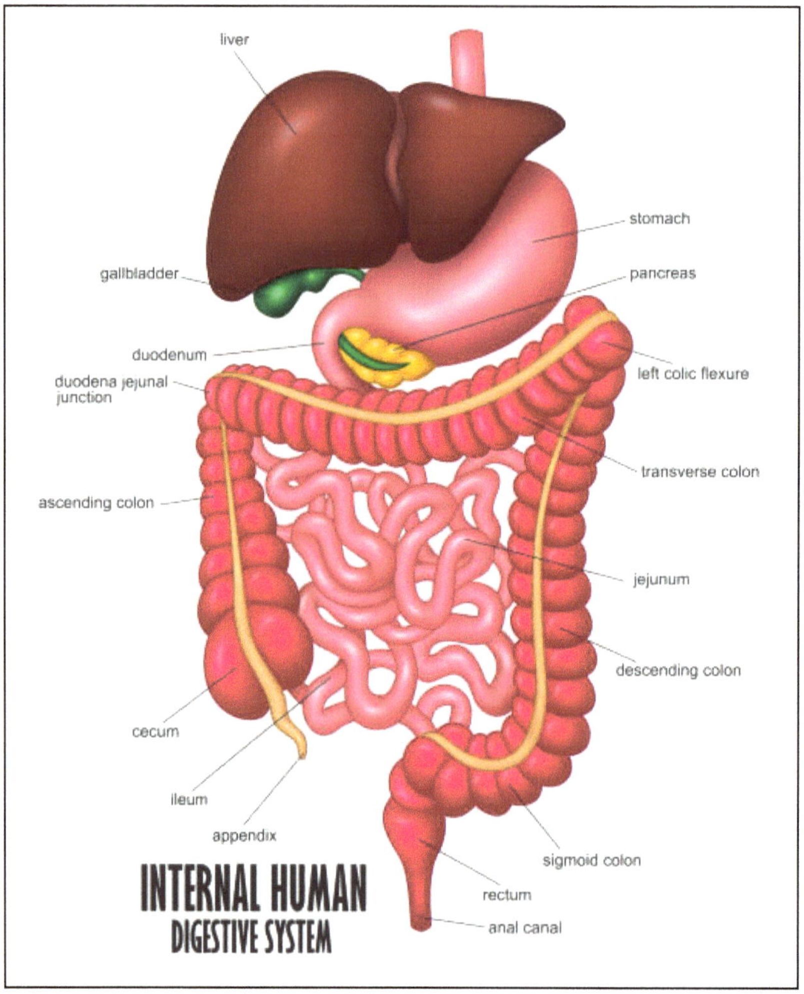

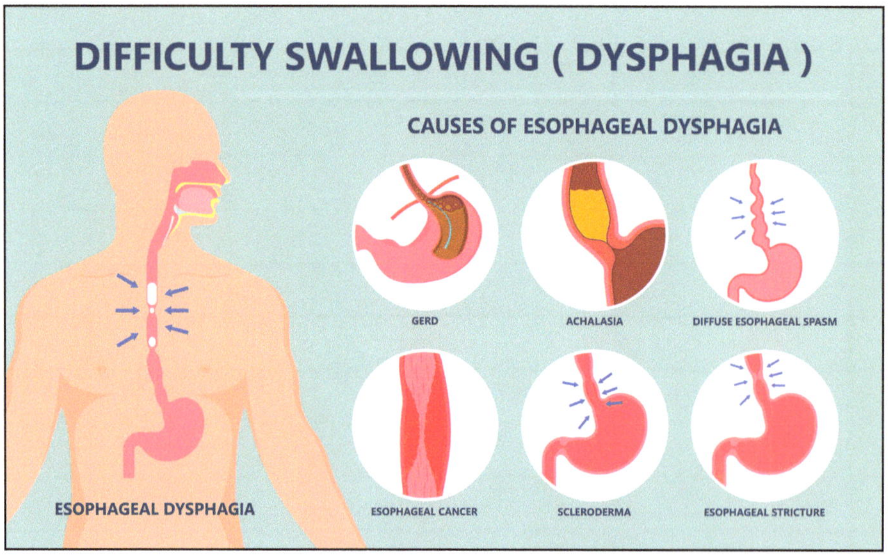

Esophageal Disorders

Eosinophilic Esophagitis: **Eosinophilic infiltration of esophageal tissue**

Sx:

PE:

Dx: Endoscopy +/- corrugated rings

____ Tx:

____

____

Pill Induced Esophagitis:

Sx: Painful swallowing, dysphagia

PE:

Dx:

____ Tx:

____

____

Infectious Esophagitis: **Seen in immunocompromised patients**

Sx: Candida = white plaques

EBV, TB, MAC, CMV = large ulcers

HSV = punched lesions

PE:

Dx:

____ Tx:

____

____

Non-Infectious Esophagitis: GERD most common etiology

Sx: Painful swallowing, heartburn, dysphagia, belching

PE:

Dx:

Tx:

Gastroesophageal Reflux Disease (GERD): Can lead to Barrett's esophagus

Sx:

PE:

Dx: EGD

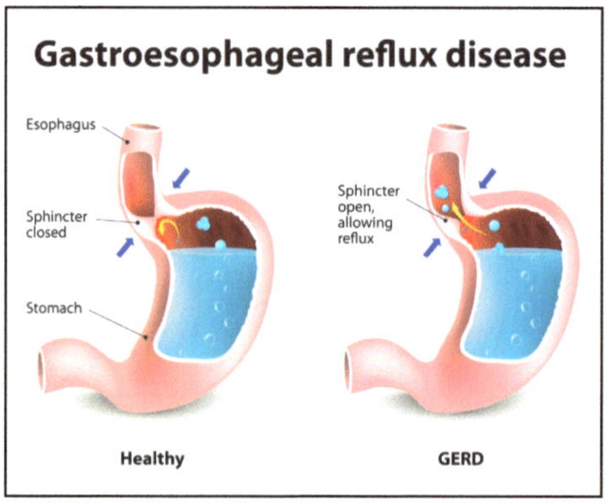

Tx:

Barrett's Esophagus: Precancerous metaplastic columnar cells

Sx:

PE:

Dx: Endoscopy with biopsy

Tx:

Mallory-Weiss Tear: **Tear in mucosa - most commonly from vomiting**

Sx:

PE:

Dx: EGD

____

____

____

Tx:

Achalasia:

Sx: Dysphagia of both solids and liquids

PE:

Dx: Swallow study with bird beak, manometry > 45mmHg

____

____

____

Tx:

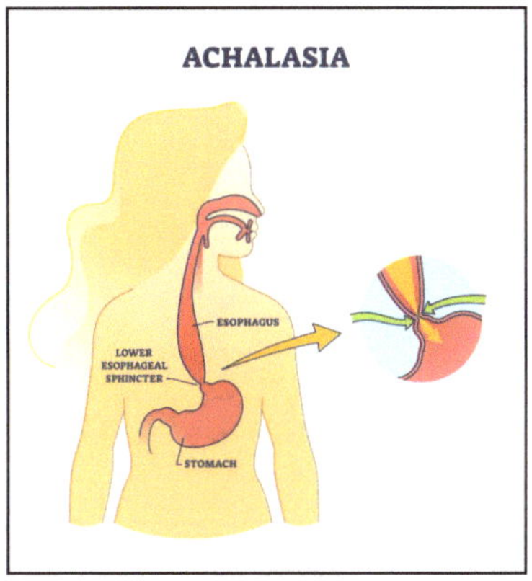

Diffuse Esophageal Spasms (DES):

Sx:

PE:

Dx: Barium swallow with corkscrew, manometry

____

____

____

Tx:

Nutcracker Esophagus: **Severe DES**

Sx:

PE:

Dx: Manometry > 180 mmHg

Tx:

Esophageal Strictures:

Sx: Dysphagia with solid foods

PE:

Dx: Endoscopy

Tx:

Esophageal (Schatzki) Ring: **Most commonly associated with sliding hiatal hernia**

Sx:

PE:

Dx: Barium esophagram

Tx:

Esophageal Varices: Portal hypertension

Sx:

PE:

Dx: Upper endoscopy

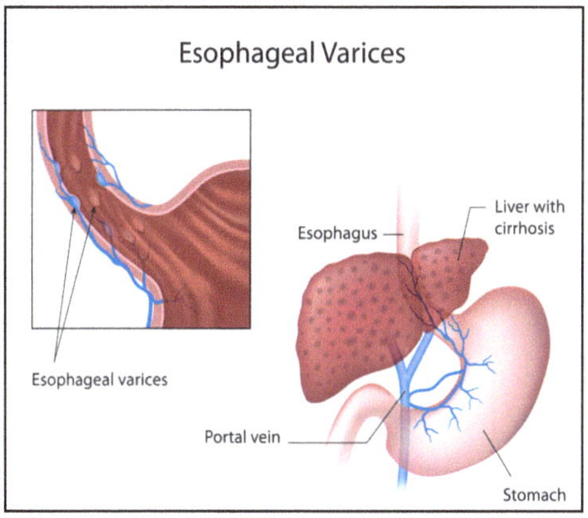

Tx:

Boerhaave's: Esophageal rupture/perforation

Sx:

PE:

Dx: Chest X-ray (initial), CT, contrast esophagram (diagnostic)

Tx:

Zenker's Diverticulum: Pharyngeal pouch

Sx: Foul odor

PE:

Dx: Barium swallow

Tx:

Gastric Disorders

Gastritis: Causes - H. pylori, autoimmune, NSAIDs

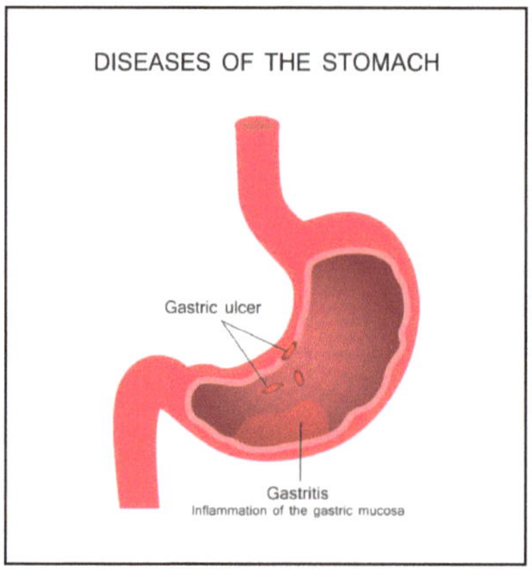

Sx:

PE:

Dx: EGD with biopsy

____

____

____

Tx:

Peptic Ulcer Disease: Causes - H. pylori, medications, Zollinger-Ellison

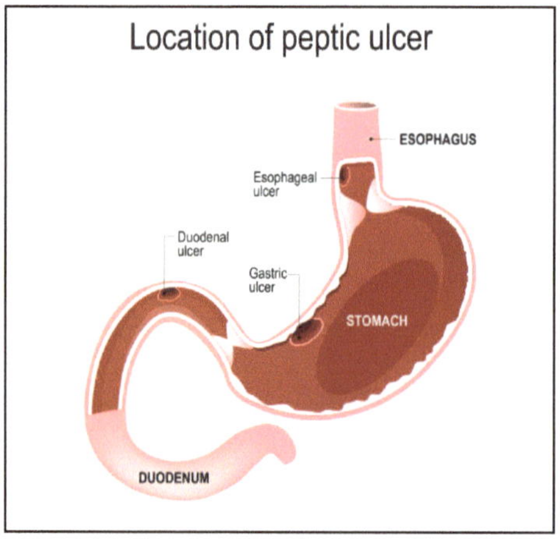

Sx:

PE:

Dx: Endoscopy (Gold Standard) +/- biopsy

____

____

____

Tx:

H. Pylori: Gram-negative bacteria

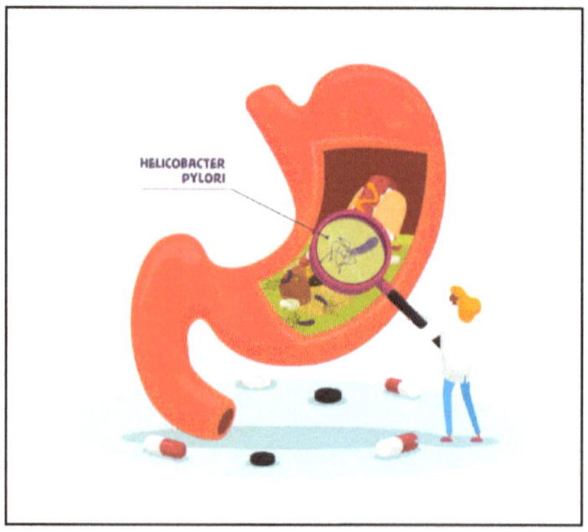

Sx:

PE:

Dx: Urea breath test, fecal antigen test, blood work

____

____

____

Tx:

Zollinger-Ellison Syndrome: **Neuroendocrine tumor that secretes gastrin**

Sx:

PE:

Dx: High gastrin levels

Tx:

Pyloric Stenosis: **Males aged 3-6 weeks**

Sx:

PE: RUQ mass - olive shaped

Dx:

Tx:

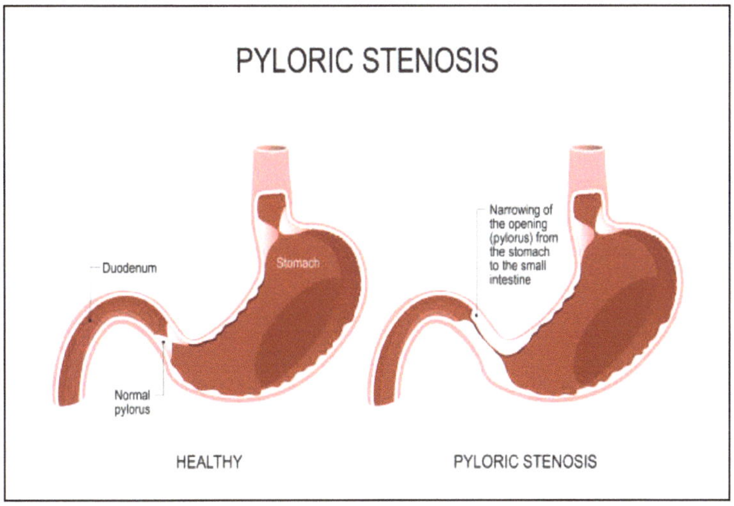

Biliary Disorders

Cholecystitis:

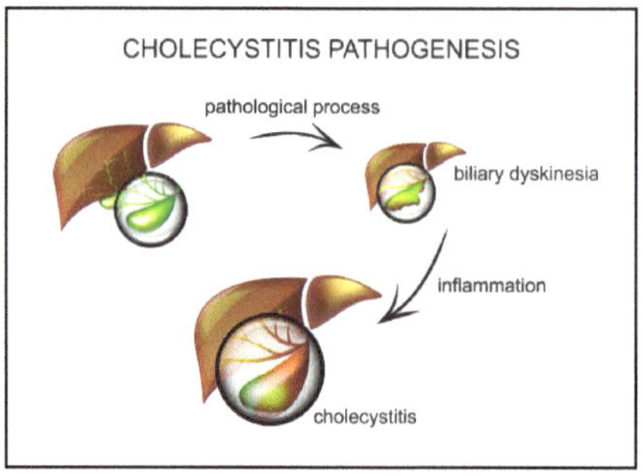

Risk Factors: Female, fat, forty, fertile

Sx:

PE: + Murphy's sign

Dx: HIDA gold standard

____

____

____

Tx:

Cholelithiasis:

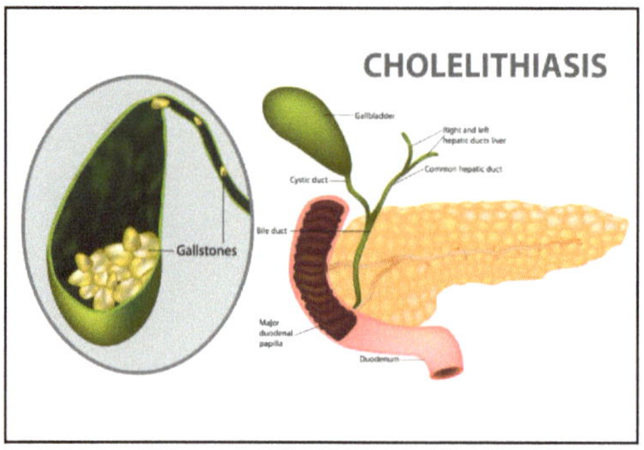

Sx: Colicky RUQ pain

PE:

Dx: US

____

____

____

Tx:

Choledocholithiasis: **Common bile duct obstruction**

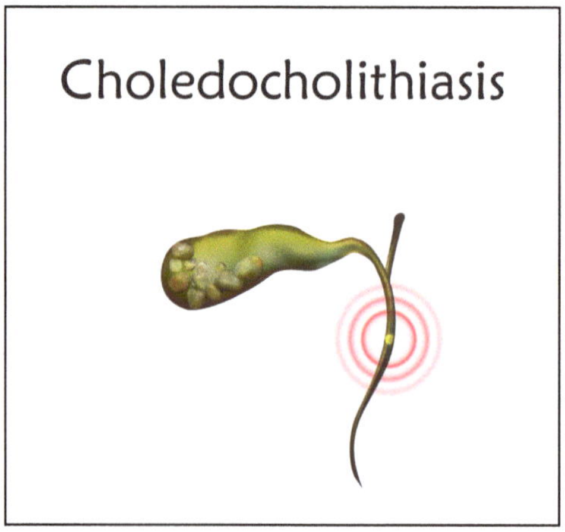

Sx:

PE:

Dx: ERCP

____

____

____

Tx:

Acute Ascending Cholangitis: Infection of biliary tree

Sx: Charcot's triad:

Reynold's pentad:

PE:

Dx: ERCP

Tx:

Primary Sclerosis Cholangitis: Chronic inflammation of liver and bile ducts

Sx:

PE:

Dx: ERCP

Tx:

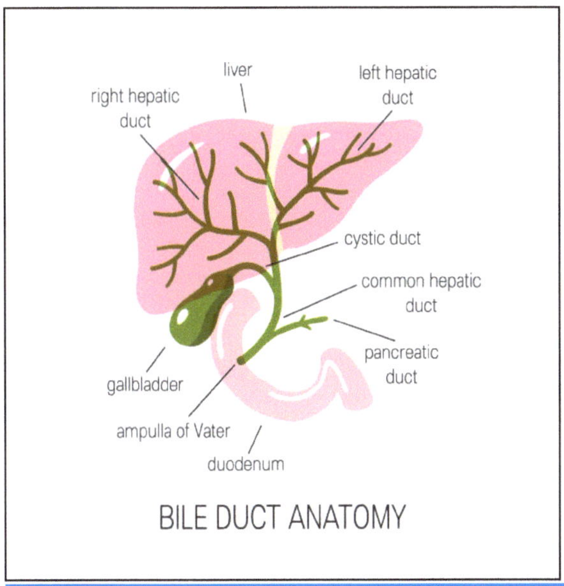

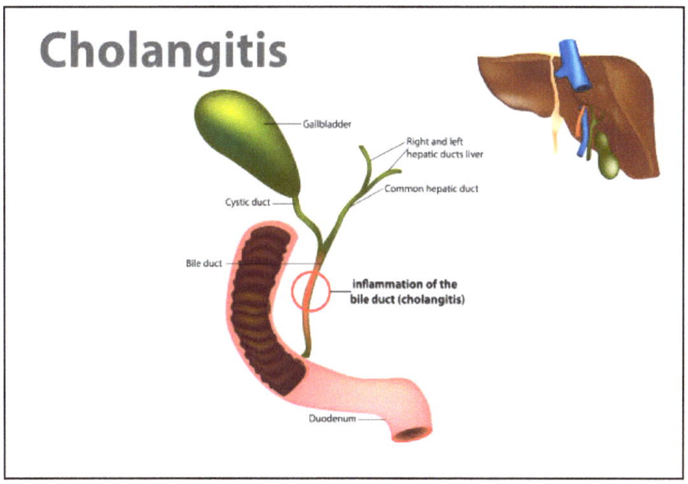

Hepatitis A: Fecal-oral

Sx:

PE:

Dx: Anti-HAV IgM

Tx:

Hepatitis B:

Sx:

PE:

Dx: Vaccinated: + Anti-HBs

Acute inf: +HBsAg +/- antiHBc IgM

Chronic: + HBsAg + Anti-HBc IgG HBeAg = infective

Hepatitis C: Blood borne

Sx:

PE:

Dx: HCV Ab

Tx:

Hepatitis D: **Only occurs with Hepatitis B**

Sx:

PE:

Dx:

Tx:

Hepatitis E: **Fecal-oral**

Sx:

PE:

Dx: IgM anti-HEV

Tx:

Autoimmune Hepatitis:

Sx: Fatigue, anorexia, abdominal pain, hepatomegaly, jaundice

PE:

Dx:

Tx:

Cirrhosis:

Sx:

PE: Ascites, caput medusa, encephalopathy

Dx: US

Tx:

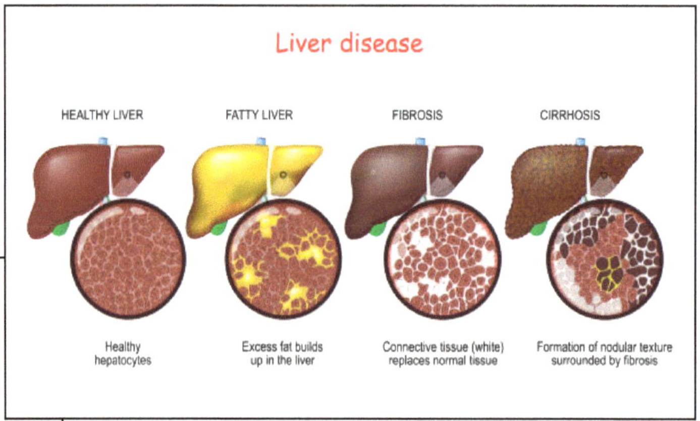

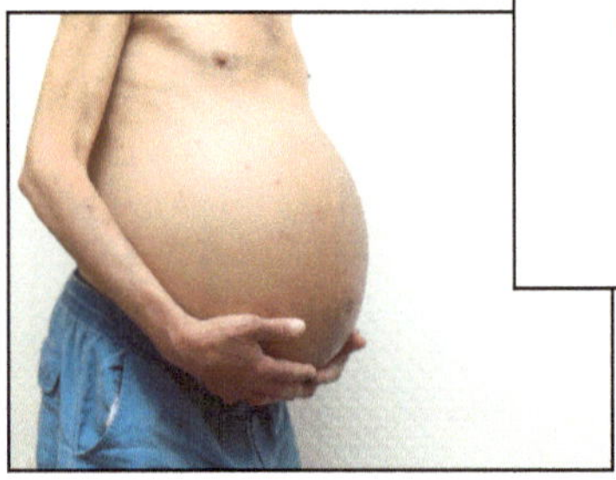

Fatty Liver Disease: Commonly associated with obesity, dyslipidemia, diabetes, and alcohol

Sx:

PE:

Dx:

Tx:

Budd-Chiari Syndrome:

Sx: Abdominal pain esophageal varices, ascites

PE:

Dx:

Tx:

Gilbert's: **Inherited disorder leading to impaired conjugation of biliribin**

Sx: Episodic jaundice with stress

PE:

Dx:

Tx:

Primary Biliary Cholangitis: **Immunologic attack**

Sx: Itching, jaundice, xanthelasma

PE:

Dx:

Tx:

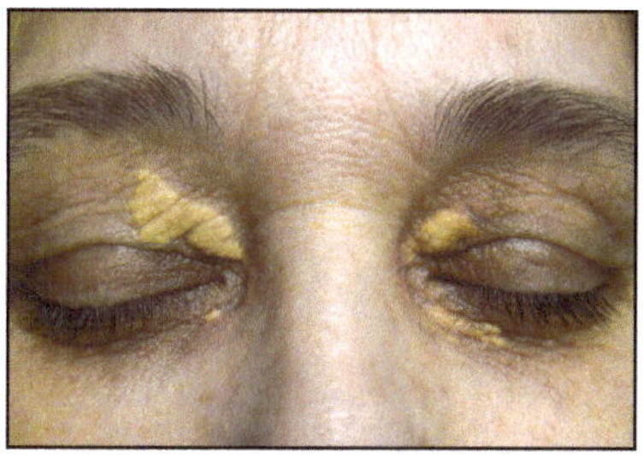

Pancreatic & Small Bowel Disorders

Pancreatitis:

Sx: Epigastric pain that radiates to the back

PE: Grey Turner's & Cullen's sign

Dx: Ranson's Criteria

____ **Tx:**

____

____

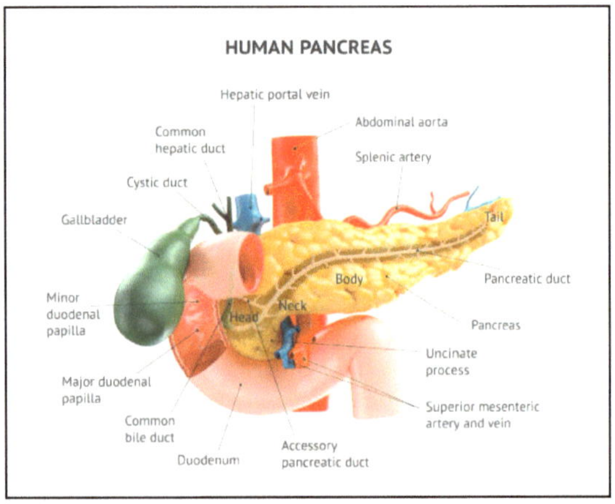

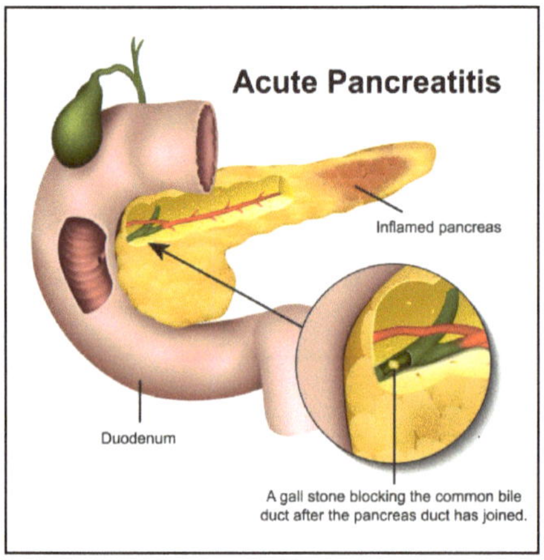

Appendicitis: **Most common cause is fecalith**

Sx: RLQ pain

PE: McBurney's, Rovsing sign, Obturator, Psoas

Dx:

____

____

____

Tx:

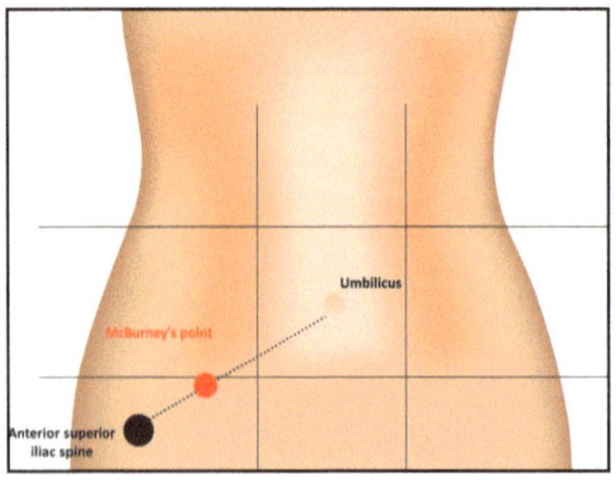

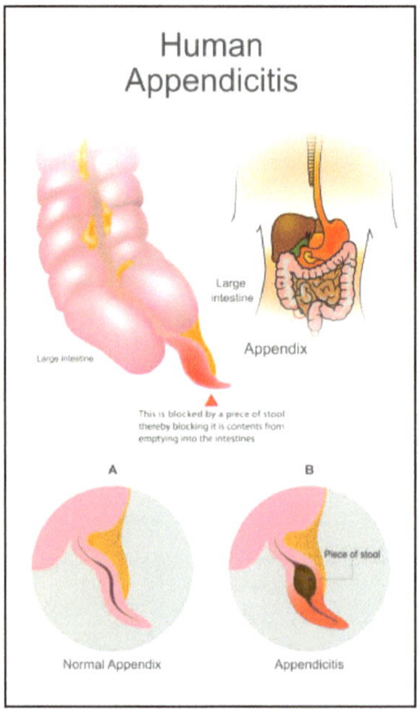

Bowel Obstruction:

Small bowel obstruction: **Post-op adhesions, high pitched bowel sounds**

Tx:

Large bowel obstruction: **Impaction, tumor**

Tx:

Dx:

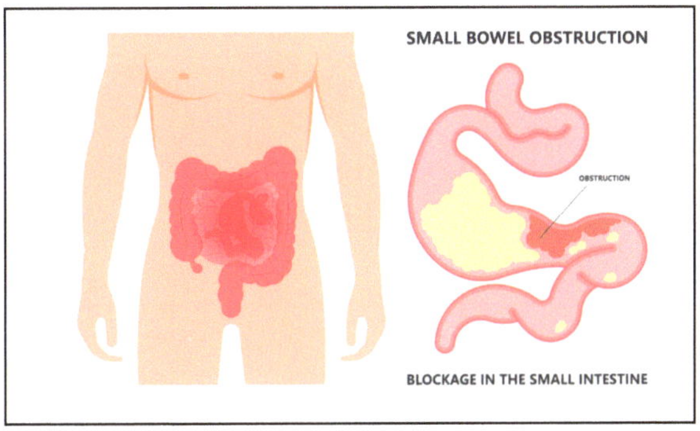

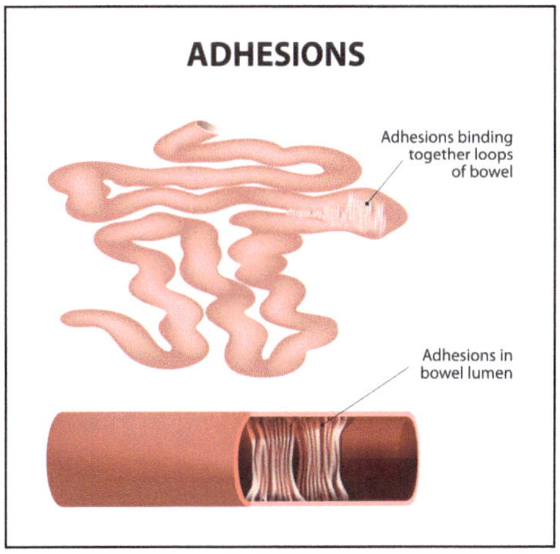

Paralytic Ileus (Ogilvie's): **Pseudo-obstructions, decreased peristalsis without obstruction**

Sx:

PE:

Dx:

Tx:

Ischemic Colitis:

Sx:

PE: Severe abdominal pain with bloody diarrhea

Dx: Colonoscopy

Tx:

Volvulus:

Sigmoid (elderly)

Midgut (infants)

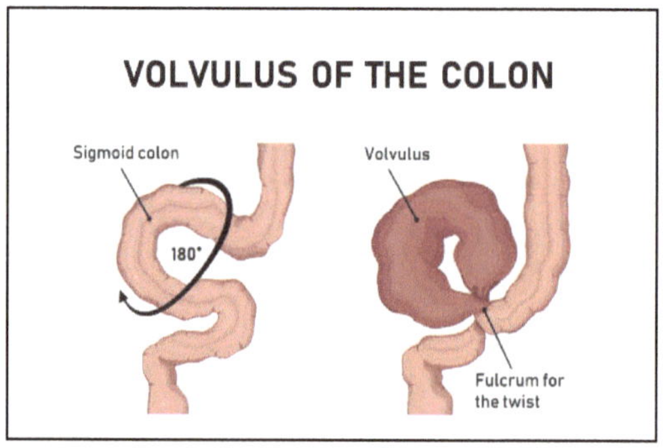

Sx:

PE:

Dx: X-ray = coffee bean
CT = whirlpool/twist

Tx:

Colorectal Disorders

Anorectal Abscess:

Sx:

PE:

Dx: Clinical

Tx:

Anorectal Fistula: Complication of deep abscess

Risk Factor: Crohn's

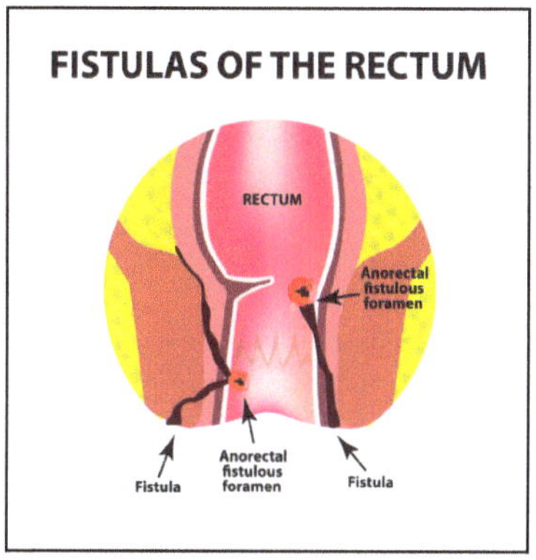

Sx: Anal discharge and pain

PE:

Dx:

Tx:

Anal Fissure: Tear distal to dentate line - most commonly posterior

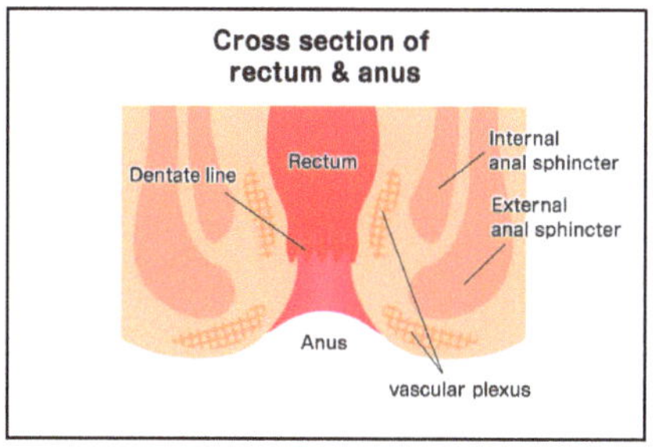

Sx: Rectal pain with bowel movement

PE:

Dx:

Tx:

Constipation: **< 2 weeks, most common causes = opiates, hypothyroidism, dehydration**

Sx:

PE:

Dx:

Tx:

Hemorrhoids: **Engorged rectal veins**

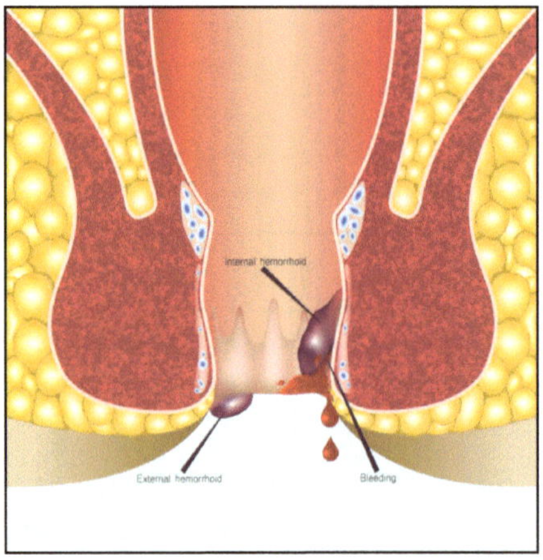

Sx: Internal = nonpainful, bleeding, pruritis
External = painful

PE:

Dx:

Tx:

Colon Polyps:

Sx: Often asymptomatic

PE:

Dx: Colonoscopy with biopsy

Tx:

Lynch Syndrome: Inherited disorder increasing risk of colon cancer

Sx:

PE:

Dx: Colonoscopy with biopsy

Tx:

Peutz-Jeghers Syndrome: Autosomal dominant, hamartomatous polyps, hyperpigmentation (lips, oral mucosa, hands)

Sx:

PE:

Dx: Colonoscopy with biopsy

Tx:

Diverticulosis: Out pouching of colon mucosa

Sx: Left lower quadrant colicky pain, painless rectal bleeding

PE:

Dx:

Tx:

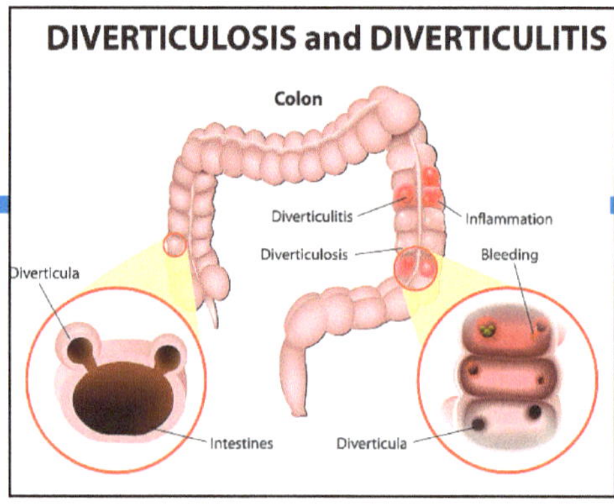

Diverticulitis:

Sx: LLQ pain, fever

PE:

Dx: CT with fat stranding, leukocytosis

Tx:

Intussusception: Telescoping of intestines

Sx: Intermittent abdominal pain, bloody stool

PE:

Dx:

Tx:

Toxic Megacolon:

Sx: Fever, abdominal pain, nausea, vomiting, rectal bleeding, bloating

PE:

Dx:

Tx:

Irritable Bowel Syndrome (IBS):

Sx:

PE:

Dx: Diagnosis of exclusion - ROME IV criteria

Tx:

Inflammatory Bowel Disease: Inflammatory, autoimmune

Ulcerative Colitis:

Sx: Bloody diarrhea, lower abdominal pain

PE:

Dx:

Tx:

Risk for cancer & toxic megacolon

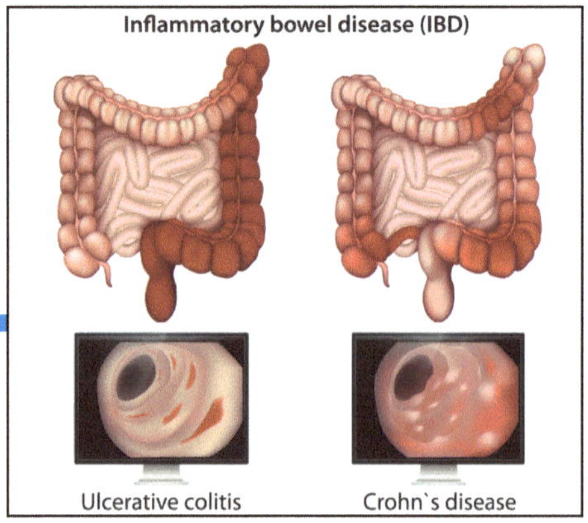

Crohn's: Mouth to anus

Sx:

PE:

Dx: Cobblestoning, skip lesions

Tx:

Risk for granuloma, fissure, fistulas

GI Neoplasms

Esophageal Cancer:

Sx: Dysphagia

PE:

Dx: EGD with biopsy

___

___

___

Tx:

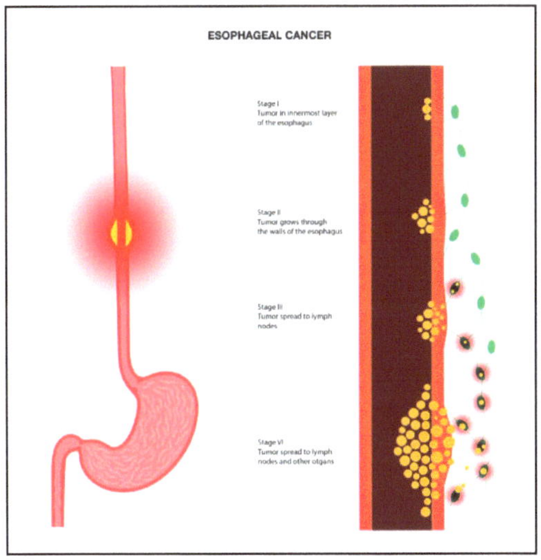

Adenocardinoma: Distal ⅓ - Barrett's esophagus precursor

Sx:

PE:

Dx:

___

___

___

Tx:

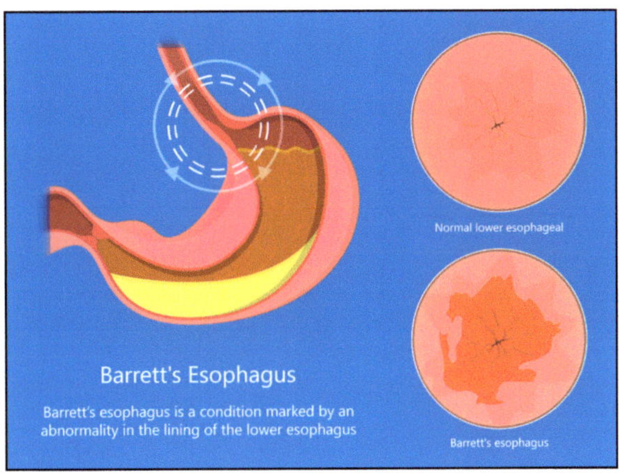

Squamous Cell Carcinoma: **Proximal 2/3**

Sx:

PE:

Dx:

Tx:

Stomach Cancer:

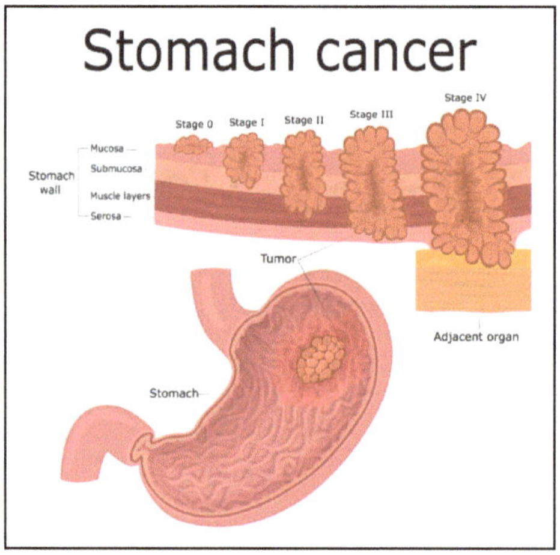

Risk Factors: H. pylori, salts, smoked meats, low fiber

Sx:

PE: Sister Mary Joseph nodule

Dx: EGD

Tx:

Hepatocellular Carcinoma: **Most common in cirrhosis**

Sx:

PE:

Dx: Alpha-fetoprotein

Tx:

Pancreatic Cancer: Head of pancreas

Sx:

PE: Courvoisier's (painless jaundice, palpable nontender gallbladder)

Dx: CT, CA 19-9

Tx:

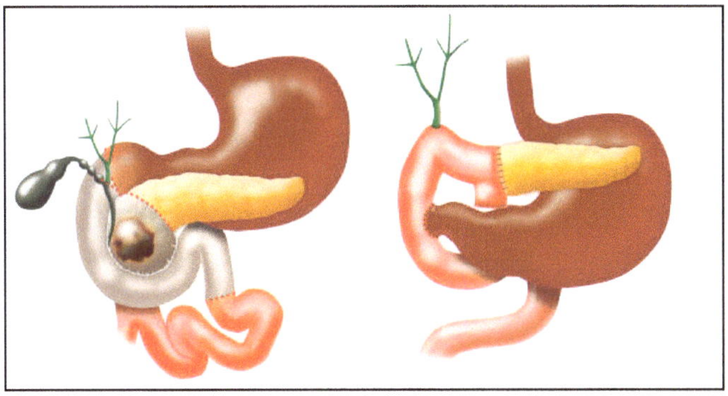

Colon Cancer: Most common adenocarcinoma

Sx: Painless rectal bleeding

PE:

Dx: Apple core lesion on barium enema, CEA

Tx:

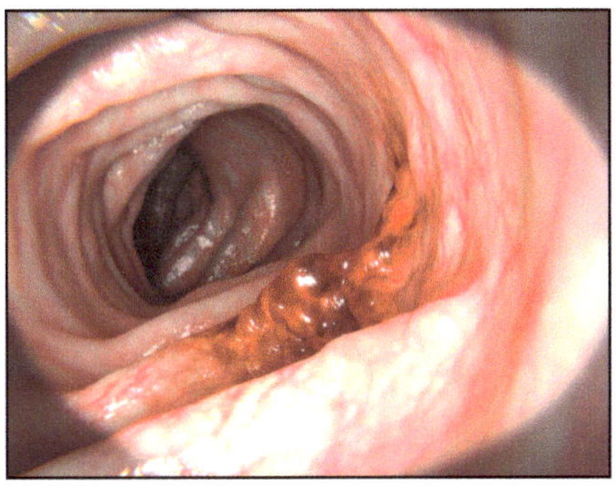

Carcinoid Syndrome: MEN Type 1 (MEN1)

Sx: Abdominal pain, weight loss, palpitations, diarrhea, flushing

PE:

Dx:

Metabolic Disorders & Misc. GI

Phenylketonuria (PKU): **Autosomal recessive**

Sx: Mental retardation, odor

PE:

Dx:

____

____

____

Tx:

Celiac: **Autoimmune triggered by gluten, villous atrophy**

Sx:

PE:

Dx: Anti-tissue transglutaminase

____

____

____

Tx:

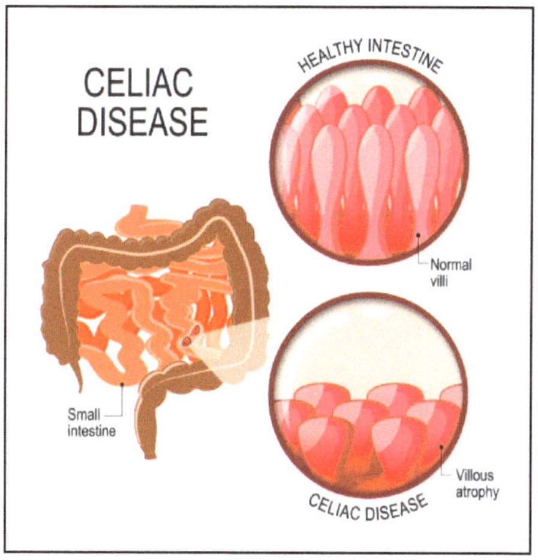

Wilson's:

Sx: Dementia, cirrhosis, Kayser-Fleischer rings, Parkinson's

PE:

Dx: High free Cu, low total serum Cu

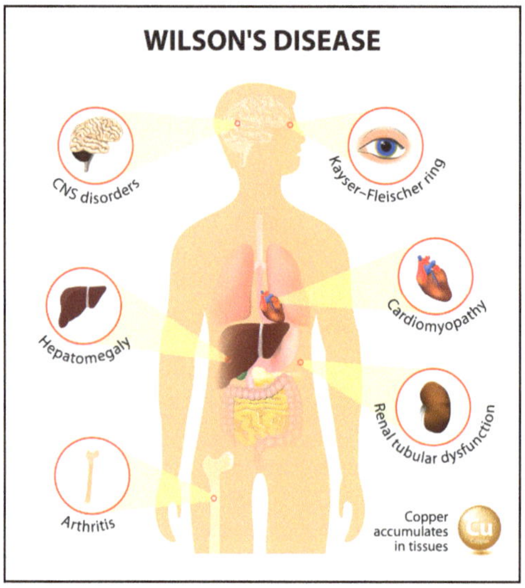

Tx:

Lactose Intolerance:

Sx:

PE:

Dx: Trial of lactose elimination

Tx:

Hernias

Indirect Inguinal Hernia: Through internal inguinal ring - lateral

Sx:

PE:

Dx:

Tx:

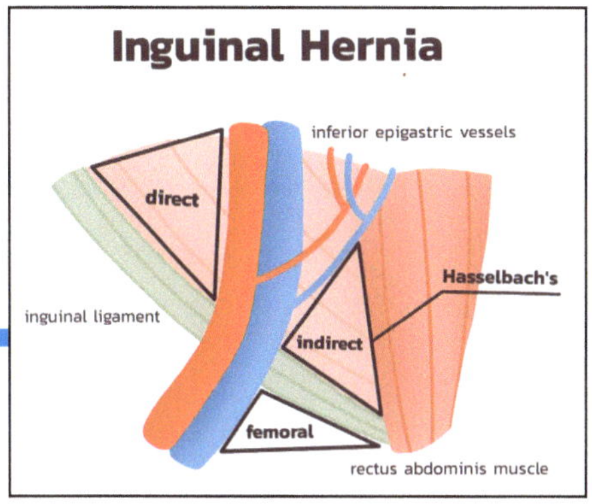

Direct Inguinal Hernia: In external inguinal ring - medial

Sx:

PE:

Dx:

Tx:

Hiatal/Diaphragmatic Hernia: Stomach through esophageal hiatus

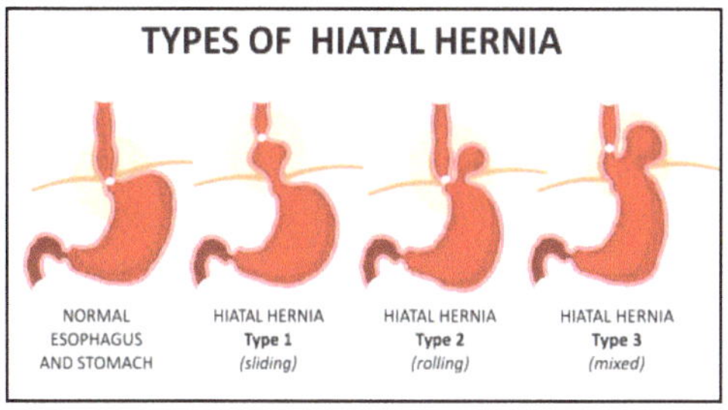

Sx:

PE:

Dx:

Tx:

Epigastric/Ventral Hernia: Often at a surgical site

Sx:

PE:

Dx:

Tx:

Umbilical Hernia: Seen at birth

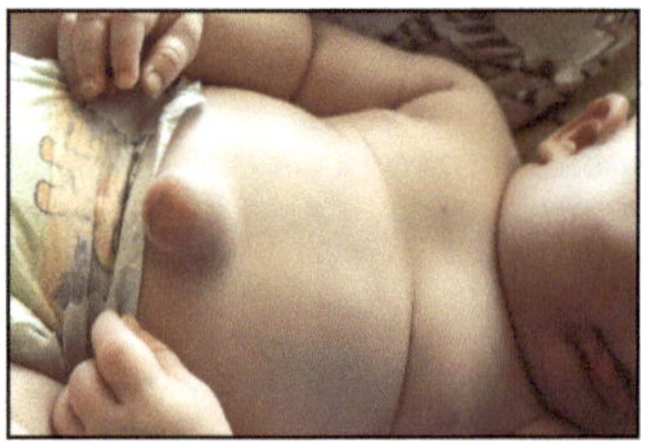

Sx:

PE:

Dx:

Tx:

Femoral Hernia: In femoral ring - risk of strangulation

Sx:

PE:

Dx:

Tx:

Diarrhea

Sx:

PE:

Dx:

S. Aureus: Picnic, egg salad

____

Tx: ______________________________

Vibrio Cholera: Shellfish

____

Tx: ______________________________

C. Perifringes: Canned food

____

Tx: ______________________________

Shigella: Daycare center, swimming, contaminated food

____

Tx: ______________________________

Salmonella: Meat, poultry, eggs, dairy

____

Tx: ______________________________

Rotavirus: Daycare center

____

Tx: ____

Norovirus: Cruise ship

____

Tx: ____

Giardia: Mountain water, foul stool

____

Tx: ____

Traveler's Diarrhea: Most common E. coli

____

Tx: ____

Typhoid:

____

Tx: ____

Cholera:

____

Tx: ____

Clostridium Difficile: Often associated with recent antibiotic use

Sx:

PE:

Dx: Stool culture

Tx:

Bariatric Surgeries

Dumping Syndrome:

Sx:

PE:

Dx:

Tx:

Vitamin Deficiencies

A: **Night vision loss, dry skin, Bitot spots in eye**

B1 (Thiamine): **Alcoholism, malnutrition, Wernicke-Korsakoff**

B2 (Riboflavin): **Glossitis, seborrheic dermatitis**

B3 (Niacin): **Dermatitis, dementia, diarrhea (Pellagra)**

B6 (Pyridoxine): **Sideroblastic anemia, weakness, insomnia, peripheral neuropathy**

B12 (Cobalamin): **Megaloblastic anemia + neurological symptoms**

C (Ascorbic acid): **Scurvy (bleeding, anemia, loose teeth)**

D: **Rickets (children), osteomalacia**

E: **Anemia, peripheral neuropathy, ataxia**

K: **Bleeding, PTT, normal bleeding time**

Vitamin Excess

A:

B3:

C:

D:

Pilonidal Disease: ***In Derm***

G6PD Deficiency: ***In Heme***

Hemochromatosis: ***In Heme***

Medications

____________________: MOA = ____________________
Indication(s)=____________________
Side Effects = ____________________
Types/ Examples = ____________________

____

____

____________________: MOA = ____________________
Indication(s)=____________________
Side Effects = ____________________
Types/ Examples = ____________________

____

____

____________________: MOA = ____________________
Indication(s)=____________________
Side Effects = ____________________
Types/ Examples = ____________________

____

____

____________________: MOA = ____________________
Indication(s)=____________________
Side Effects = ____________________
Types/ Examples = ____________________

____

____

____________________: MOA = ____________________
Indication(s)=____________________
Side Effects = ____________________
Types/ Examples = ____________________

____

____

Medications

______________: MOA = ______________

Indication(s)=______________

Side Effects = ______________

Types/ Examples = ______________

____

____

______________: MOA = ______________

Indication(s)=______________

Side Effects = ______________

Types/ Examples = ______________

____

____

______________: MOA = ______________

Indication(s)=______________

Side Effects = ______________

Types/ Examples = ______________

____

____

______________: MOA = ______________

Indication(s)=______________

Side Effects = ______________

Types/ Examples = ______________

____

____

______________: MOA = ______________

Indication(s)=______________

Side Effects = ______________

Types/ Examples = ______________

____

____

Musculoskeletal/Ortho/Rheumatology

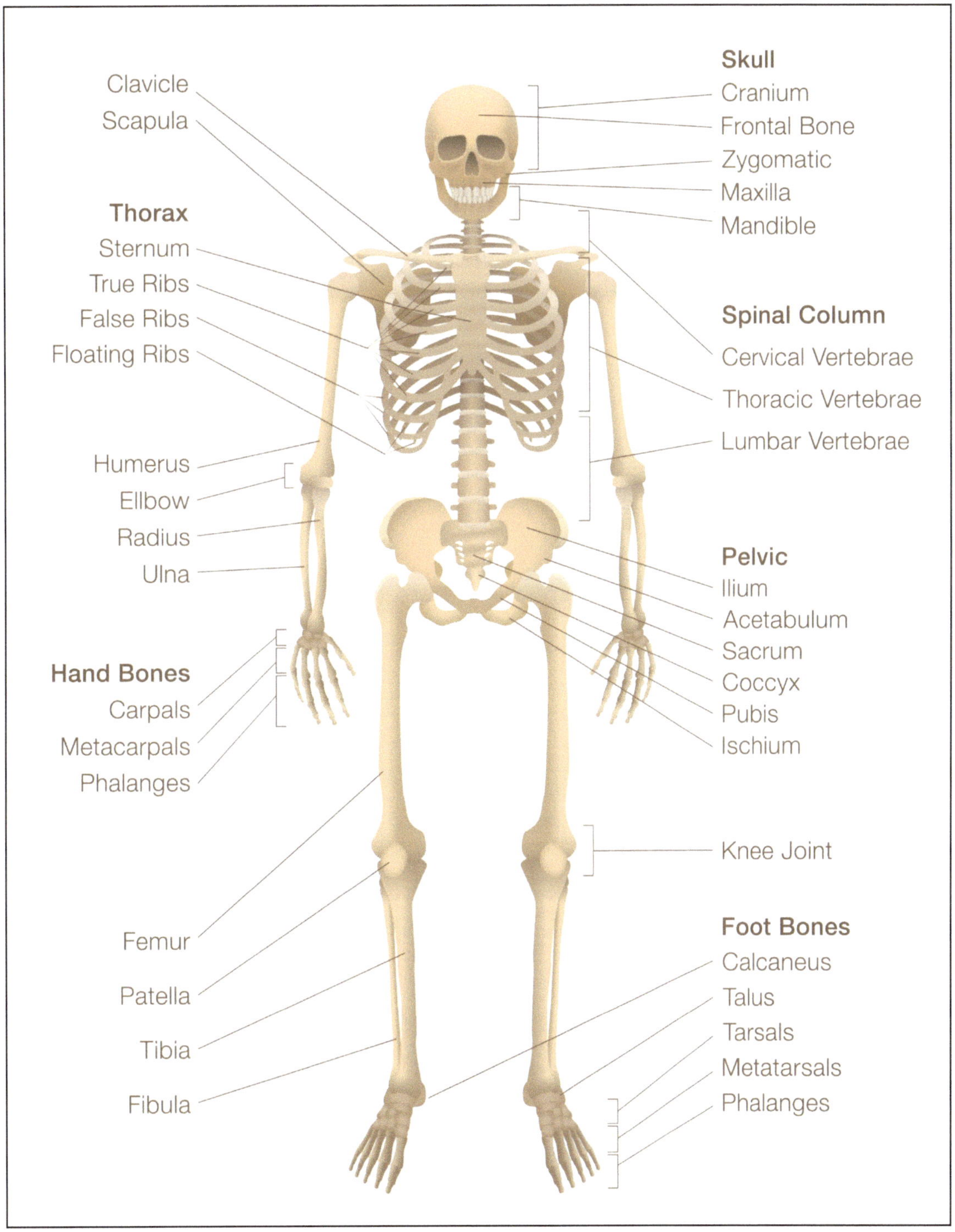

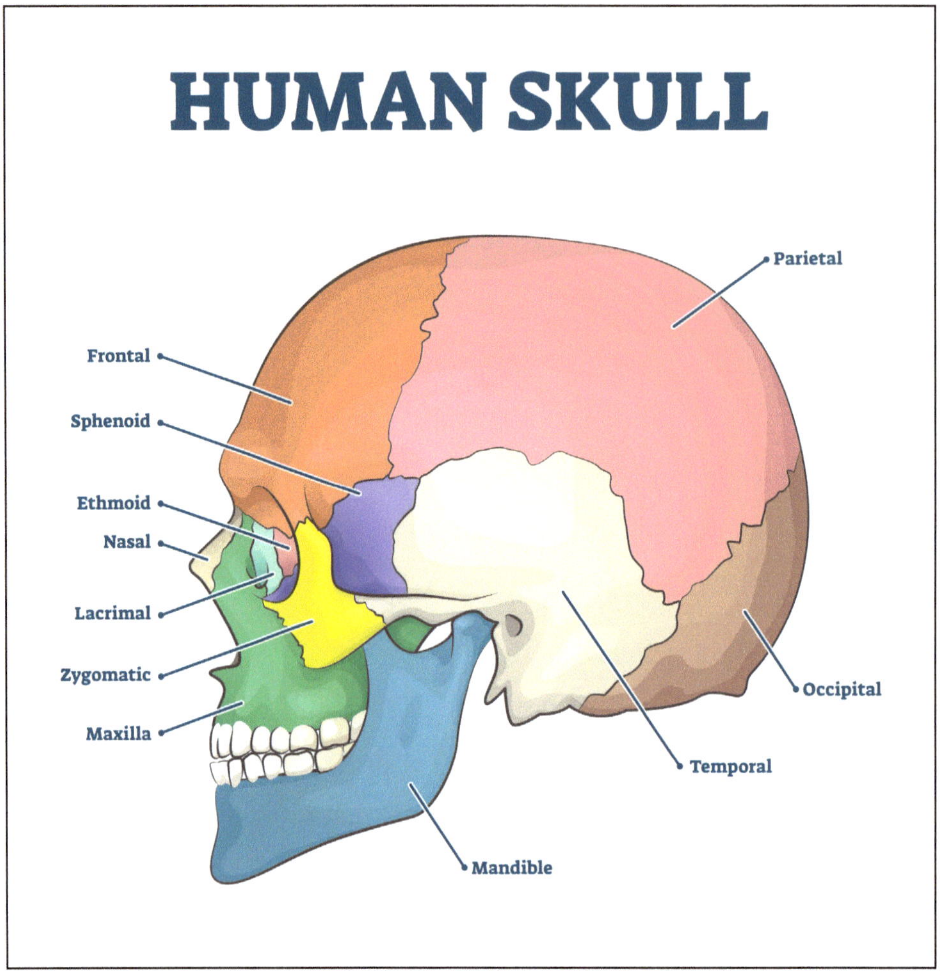
HUMAN SKULL
Parietal
Frontal
Sphenoid
Ethmoid
Nasal
Lacrimal
Zygomatic
Maxilla
Occipital
Temporal
Mandible

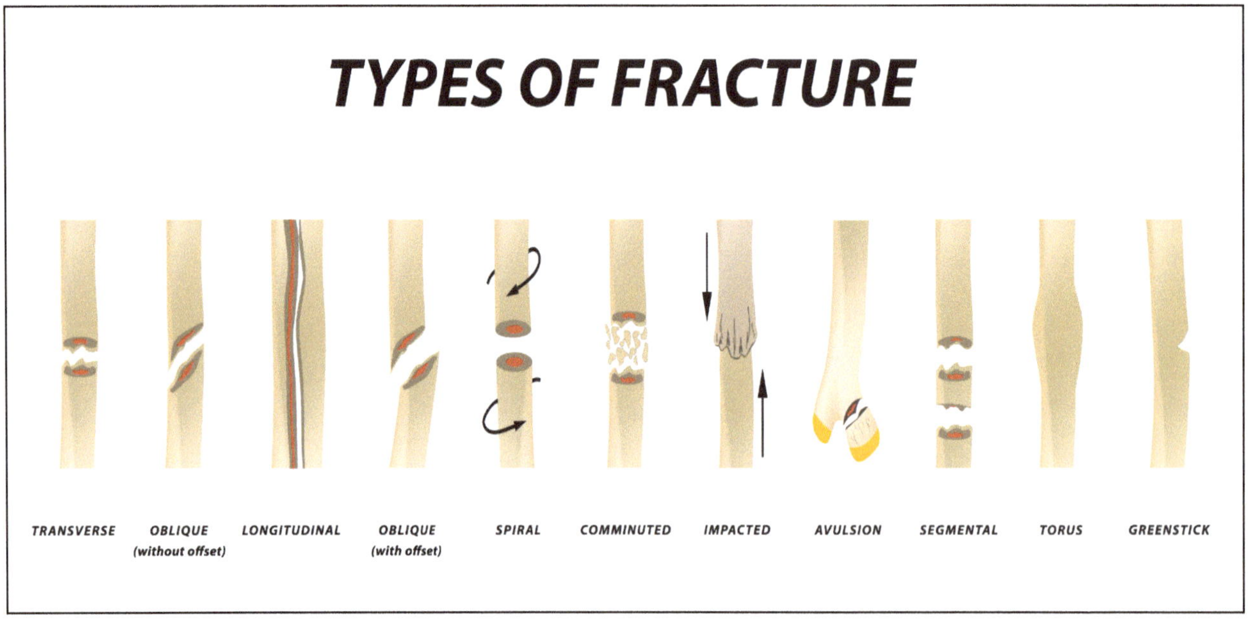
TYPES OF FRACTURE
TRANSVERSE
OBLIQUE (without offset)
LONGITUDINAL
OBLIQUE (with offset)
SPIRAL
COMMINUTED
IMPACTED
AVULSION
SEGMENTAL
TORUS
GREENSTICK

Disorders of the Elbow & Forearm

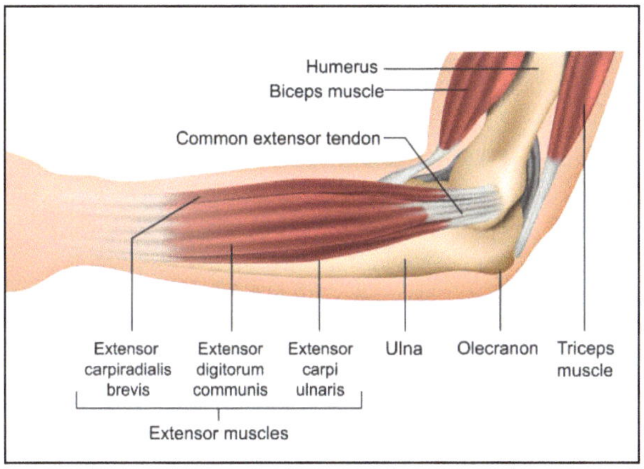

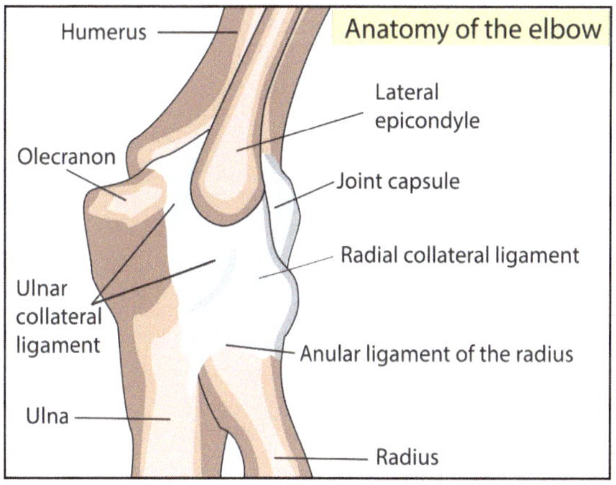

Elbow Dislocation: **Most common is posterior dislocation**

Sx: In flexion

PE:

Dx: X-ray

Tx:

Olecranon Bursitis: **Swelling from overuse**

Sx: Pain at the site of the bursa

PE: Tenderness to palpation, decreased range of motion

Dx:

Tx:

Biceps Tendonitis: **Caused from overuse**

Sx: Pain at bicipital groove

PE:

Dx: Yergason

Tx:

Biceps Tendon Rupture: **Usually trauma**

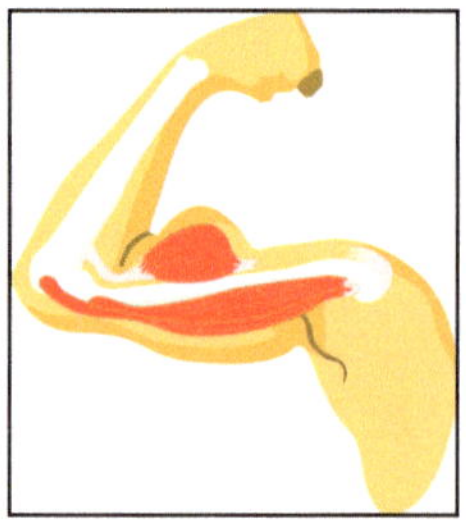

Sx: Sudden sharp pain, sometimes a "pop" sound

PE: Popeye deformity

Dx:

Tx:

Medial Epicondylitis: **Golfer's elbow**

Sx: Elbow pain during or following flexion

PE: Pain with resisted forearm pronation or wrist flexion

Dx:

Tx:

Lateral Epicondylitis: **Tennis elbow**

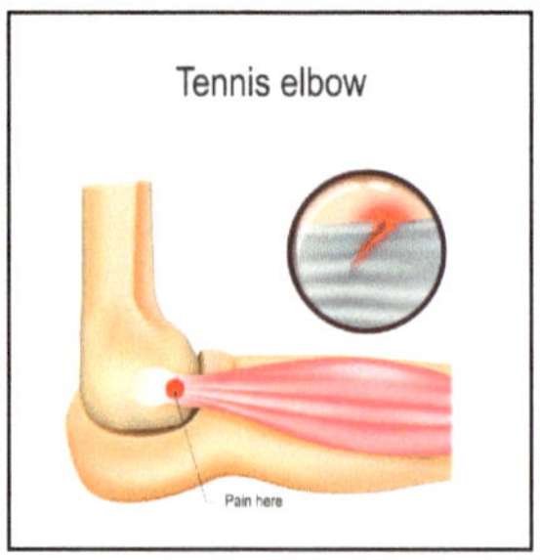

Sx: Pain with extension

PE: Pain during resisted wrist and digit extension

Dx:

Tx:

Elbow & Supracondylar Fractures:

Sx:

PX:

Dx: X-ray with anterior fat pad sign

Sail sign = kids

Radial head or proximal ulnar = adults

Tx:

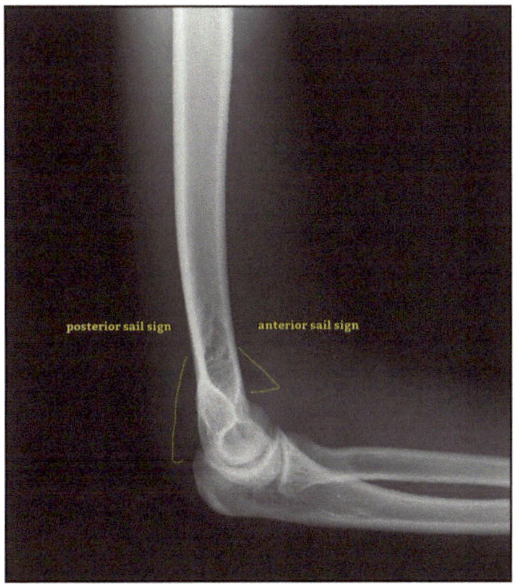

Radial Head Fracture: Most common in kids with FOOSH

Sx: Localized swelling, tender, decreased motion

PE:

Dx: X-ray

Tx:

Nightstick Fracture: **Isolated fracture of ulna**

Sx:

PE:

Dx: X-ray

Tx:

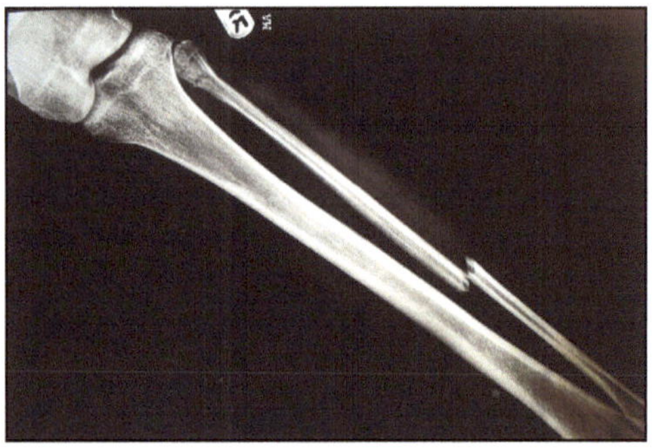

Monteggia Fracture: **Proximal ulnar fracture & radial head dislocation**

Sx: May have swelling, deformity, movement may cause pain

PE:

Dx: X-ray

Tx:

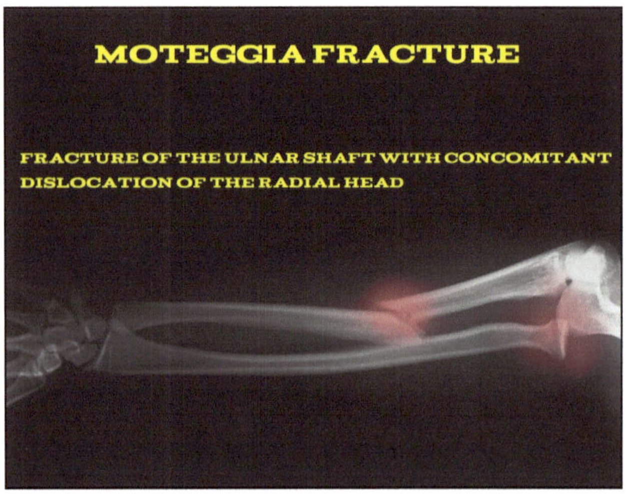

Galeazzi Fracture: Distal radial fracture & radioulnar dislocation

Sx:

PX:

Dx: X-ray

Tx:

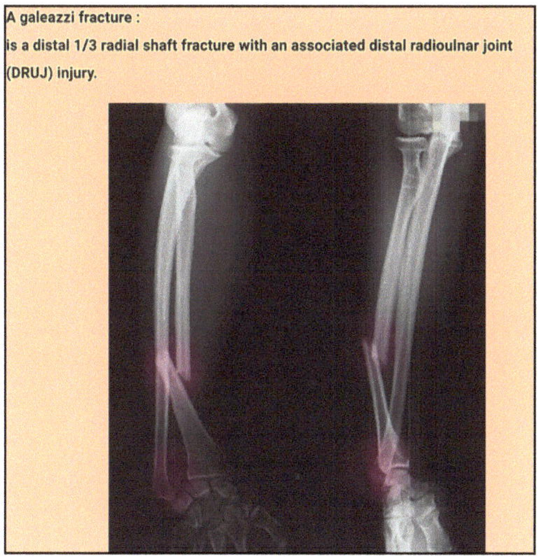

Cubital Tunnel Syndrome: Ulnar nerve compression at medial epicondyle

Sx: Pain, possible decreased grip strength

PE:

Dx: Tinel's

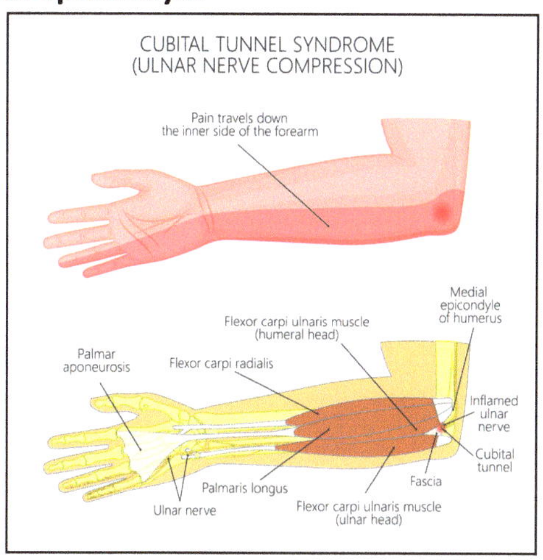

Tx:

Disorders of the Wrist & Hand

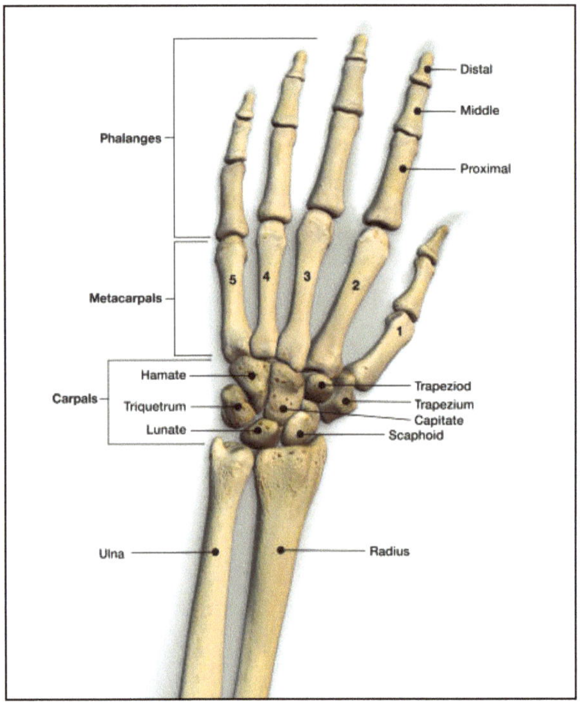

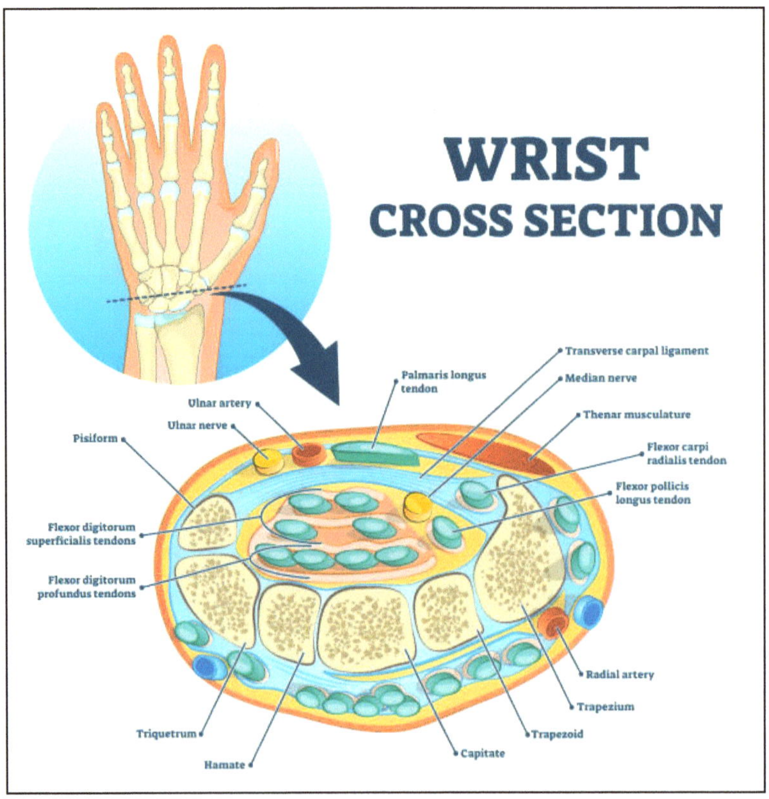

Scaphoid Fracture: FOOSH

Sx: Snuffbox tenderness, risk of avascular necrosis

PE:

Dx: X-ray = may not show up **MRI = definitive**

Repeat X-ray

Tx:

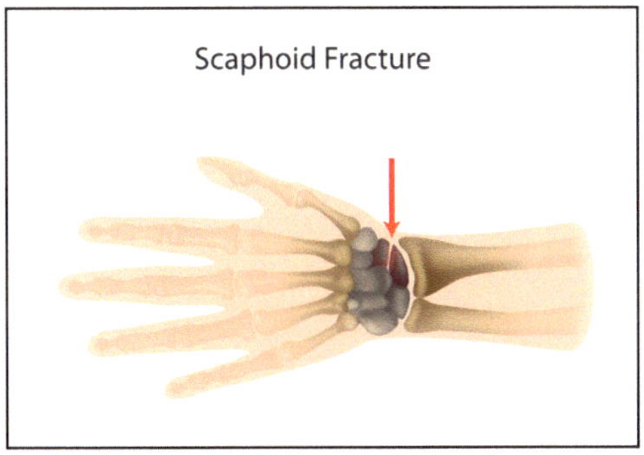

Boxer Fracture:

Sx: 5th metacarpal fracture, often punching injury

PE: Check for scissoring of fingers

Dx:

Tx:

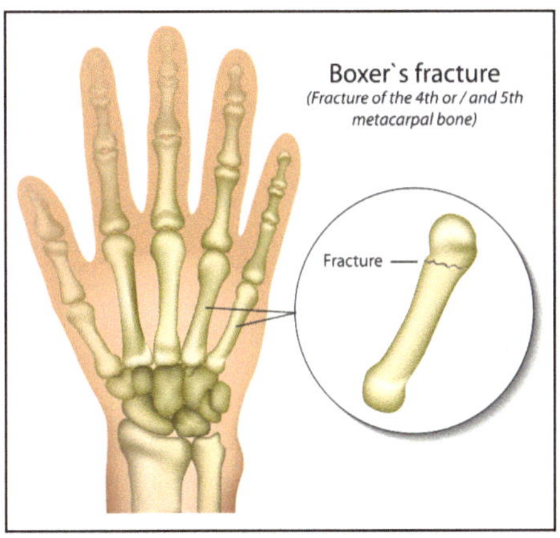

Bennett Fracture: **Usually due to axial force**

Sx: Partial fracture of 1st metacarpal

PE:

Dx: X-ray (oblique view)

______________________________________ **Tx:**

____

____

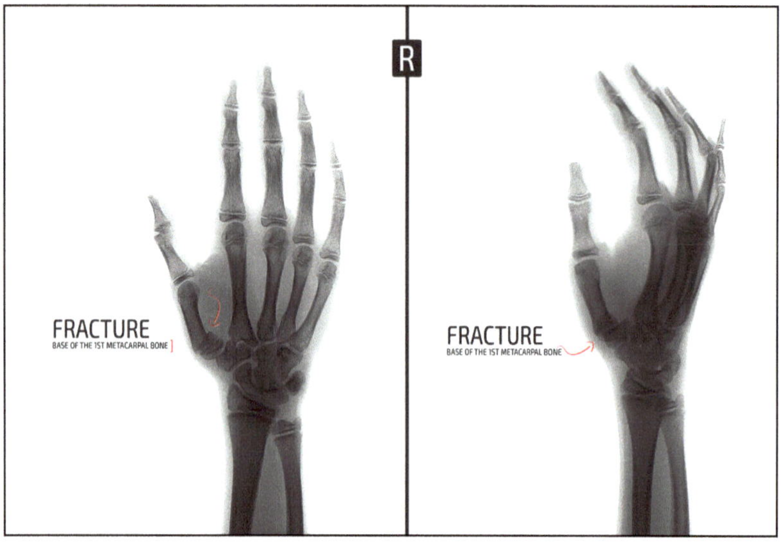

Rolando Fracture: **Prognosis worse than Bennett fracture**

Sx: Complete fracture of the 1st metacarpal, comminuted, intra-articular

PE:

Dx: X-ray (oblique view)

______________________________________ **Tx:**

____

____

DeQuervain's Tenosynovitis: Often from repetitive use

Sx: Inflammation of tendon sheath at thumb MCP

PE:

Dx: Finkelstein

Tx:

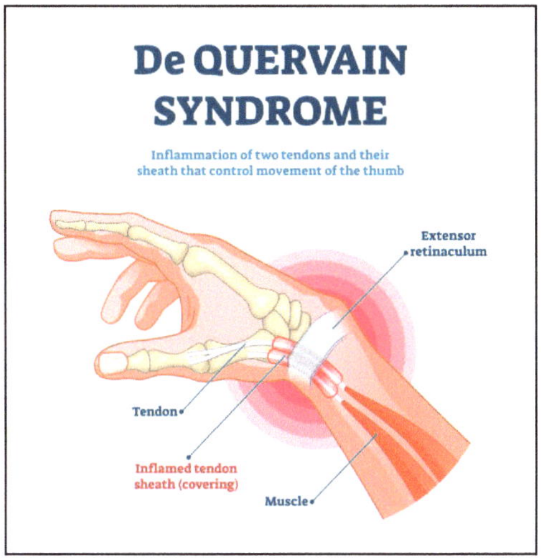

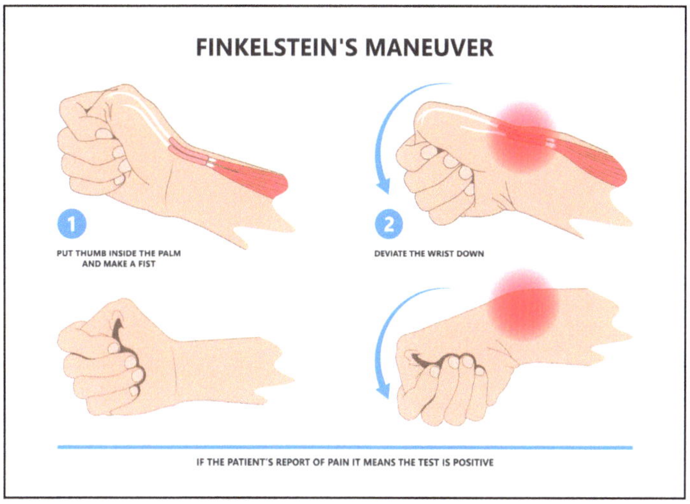

Gamekeeper's Thumb (Skier's): Ulnar collateral ligament injury, ulnar aspect of thumb

Sx: Pain with abduction, laxity with valgus stress, local swelling & bruising

PE:

Dx: X-ray or MRI

Tx:

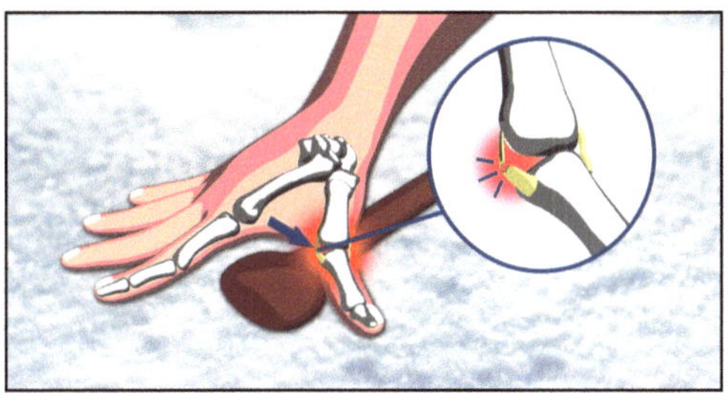

Carpal Tunnel Syndrome: Compression of median nerve at wrist, overuse injury, pregnancy can be a risk factor

Sx: Early = numbness, tingling   Late = thenar wasting

PE:

Dx: (+) Tinel, (+) Phalen

Tx:

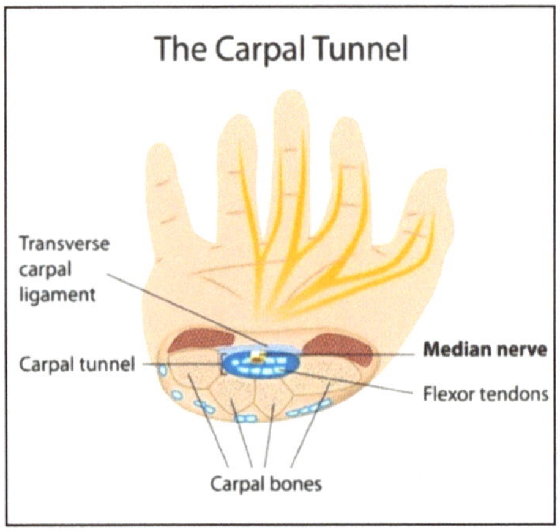

Colles' Fracture: Distal radius fracture, dorsal displacement of distal radius fragment, FOOSH (Outward)

Smith's Fracture: Distal radius fracture, palmar displacement of distal radius fragment, FOOSH (Inward)

Sx:

PE:

Dx: X-ray, assess for deformity and neurovascular compromise

Tx:

Mallet Finger: Jam injury leading to flexed DIP

Sx: Joint tenderness, swelling

PE: Cannot extend DIP

Dx:

______________________________ Tx:

____

____

Boutonniere Deformity:

Sx: Joint pain, swelling, co-occurring with rheumatoid arthritis

PE: PIP flexed, DIP extended

Dx:

______________________________ Tx:

____

____

Swan Neck Deformity:

Sx: Seen in advanced RA

PE: DIP hyperflexion with PIP hyperextension

Dx:

______________________________ Tx:

____

____

Trigger Finger: Flexor tendon locked in flexed position due to inflammation and thickening

Sx: Cannot fully extend finger, usually episodic, usually at MCP joint

PE:

Dx:

Tx:

Dupuytren's Contracture: Fibrosis of connective tissue leading to flexed PIP

Sx: Palmar skin changes with nodule, peritendinous cords

PE: PIP joint contracture

Dx:

Tx:

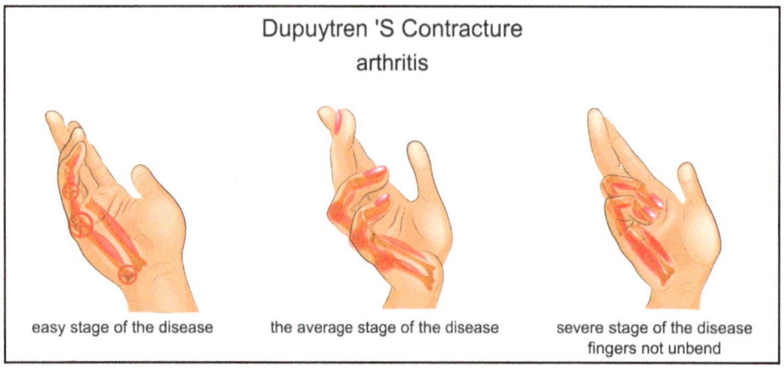

Felon: Abscess to distal finger

Sx: Acute infection of pulp space in fingertip, pain, fluctuant area and edema

PE:

Dx:

Tx:

Paronychia:

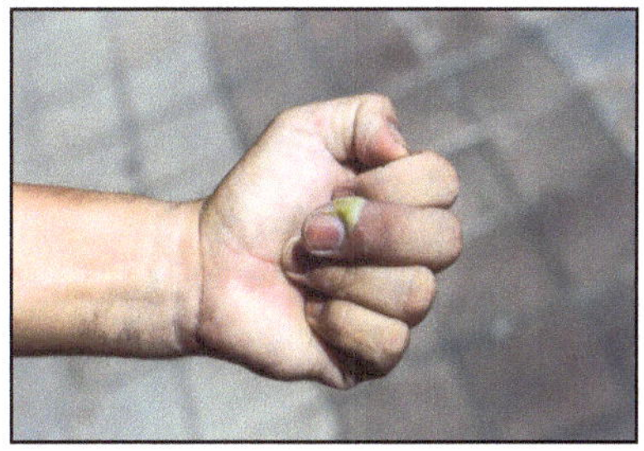

Sx: Pain, swelling, drainage

PE:

Dx:

Tx:

Finger Fractures:

Sx: Pain, swelling, bruising

PE:

Dx: X-ray

Tx:

Flexor Tenosynovitis:

Sx:

PE: Kanavel's sign

Dx:

Tx:

Kanavel's sign

Disorders of the Shoulder

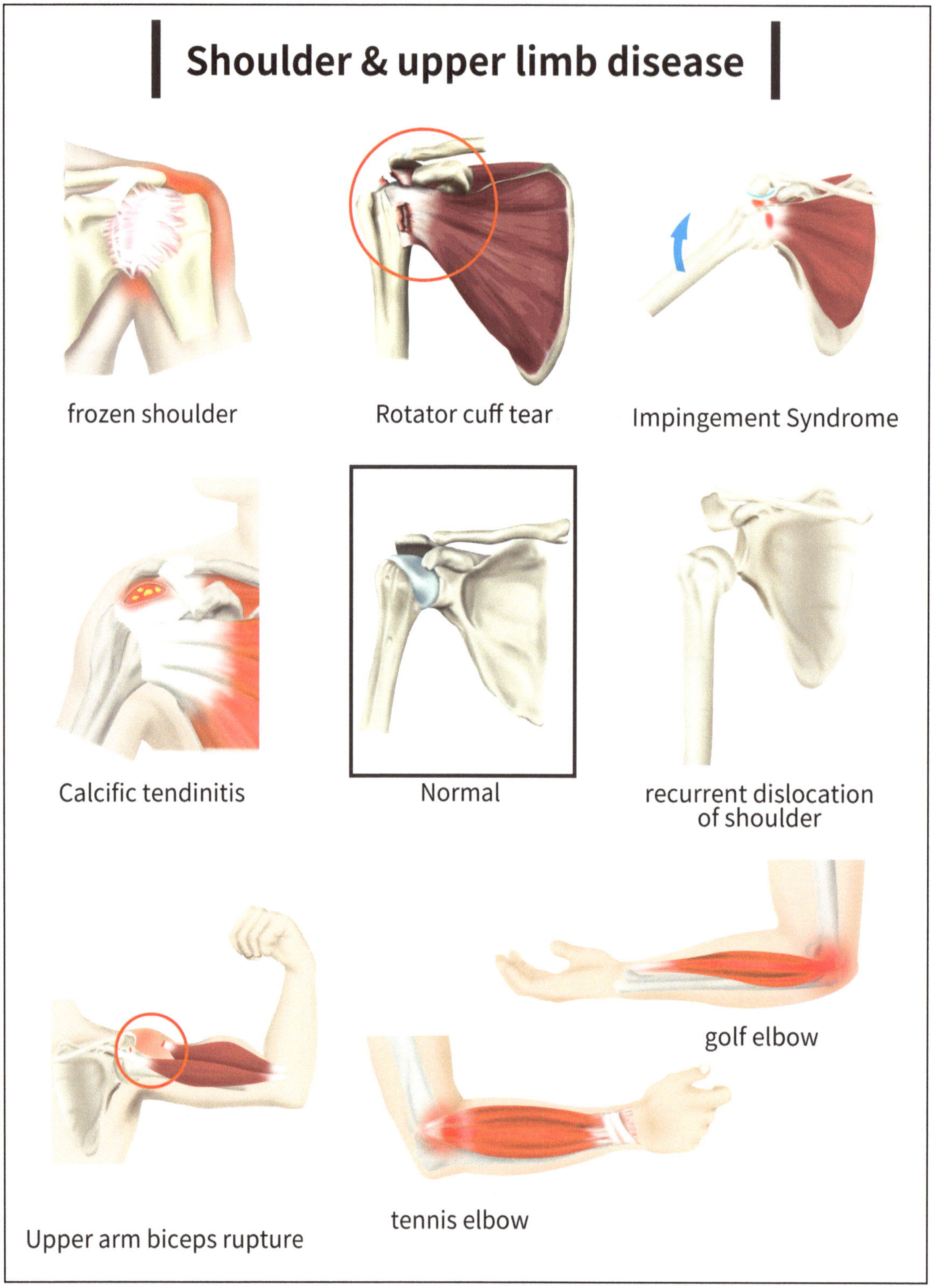

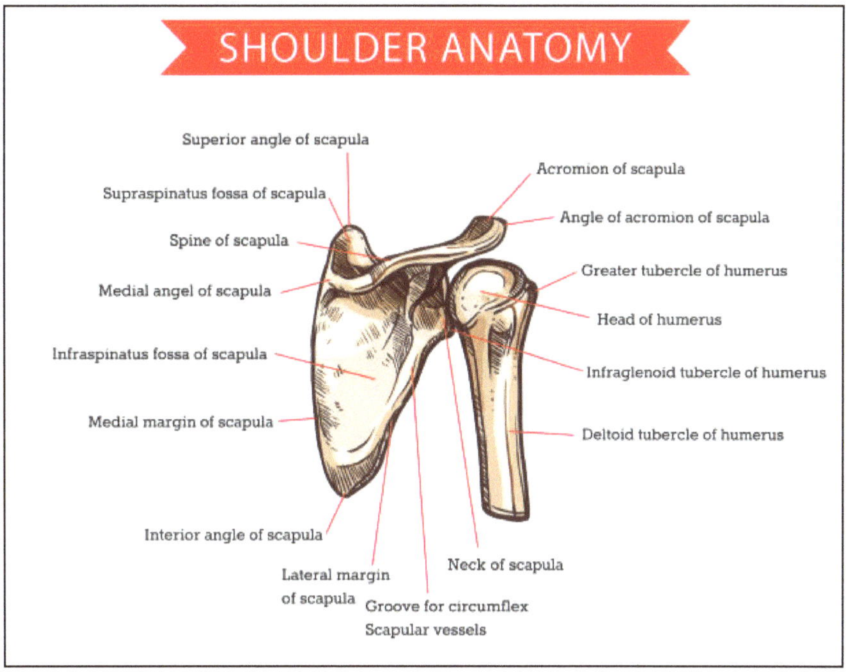
SHOULDER ANATOMY
Superior angle of scapula
Supraspinatus fossa of scapula
Spine of scapula
Medial angel of scapula
Infraspinatus fossa of scapula
Medial margin of scapula
Interior angle of scapula
Lateral margin of scapula
Groove for circumflex Scapular vessels
Neck of scapula
Acromion of scapula
Angle of acromion of scapula
Greater tubercle of humerus
Head of humerus
Infraglenoid tubercle of humerus
Deltoid tubercle of humerus

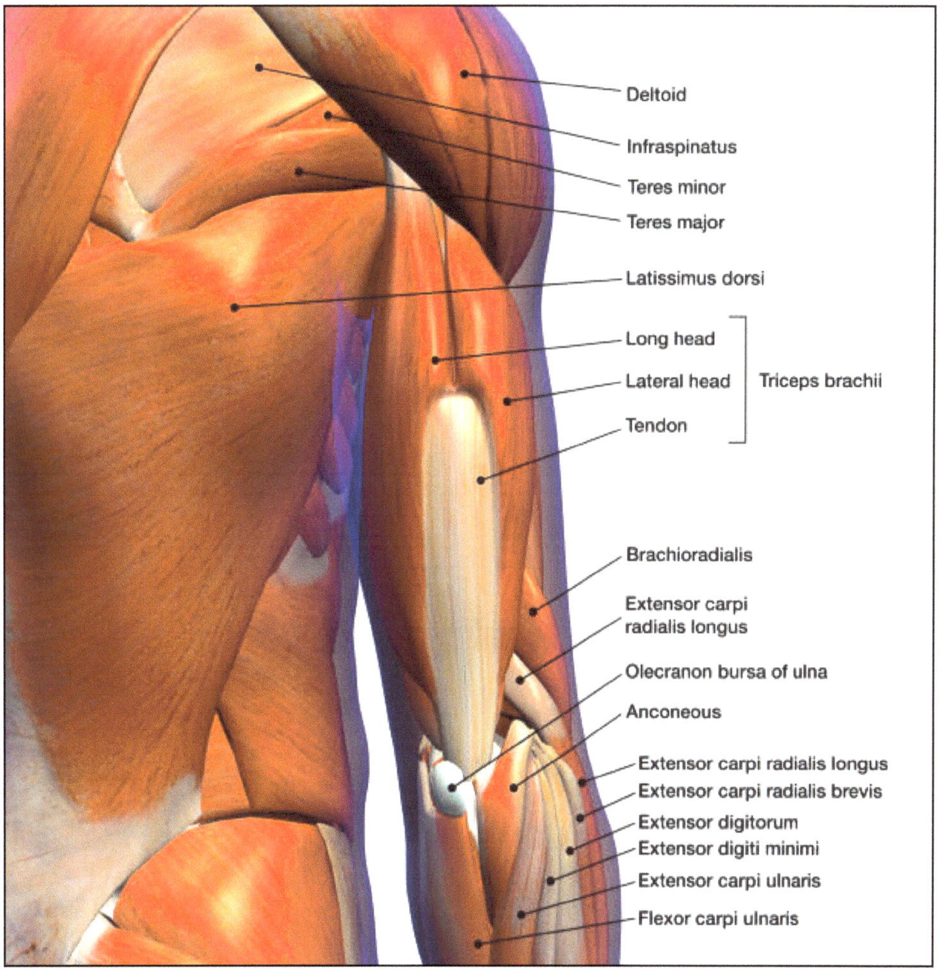
Deltoid
Infraspinatus
Teres minor
Teres major
Latissimus dorsi
Long head
Lateral head
Tendon
Triceps brachii
Brachioradialis
Extensor carpi radialis longus
Olecranon bursa of ulna
Anconeous
Extensor carpi radialis longus
Extensor carpi radialis brevis
Extensor digitorum
Extensor digiti minimi
Extensor carpi ulnaris
Flexor carpi ulnaris

Shoulder Fracture: Most common elderly

Sx: Pain

PE:

Dx: X-ray

Tx:

Bankart Lesion: When glenoid labrum is disrupted with dislocation *associated with SLAP lesion

Sx: Pain

PE:

Dx: X-ray

Tx:

Hill-Sachs Lesion: Cortical depression of humoral head made by glenoid rim

*seen in 35-40% of anterior shoulder dislocations

Sx: Pain

PE:

Dx: X-ray

Tx:

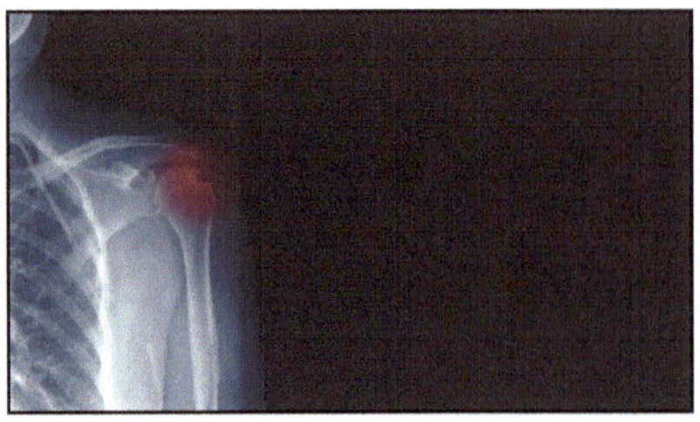

Shoulder Dislocation: Most commonly anterior

Sx: Abducted, externally rotated arm - (possible axillary nerve injury)

PE:

Dx: X-ray

Tx:

Clavicle Fracture:

Sx: Swelling, pain with movement

PE:

Dx: AP X-ray

Tx:

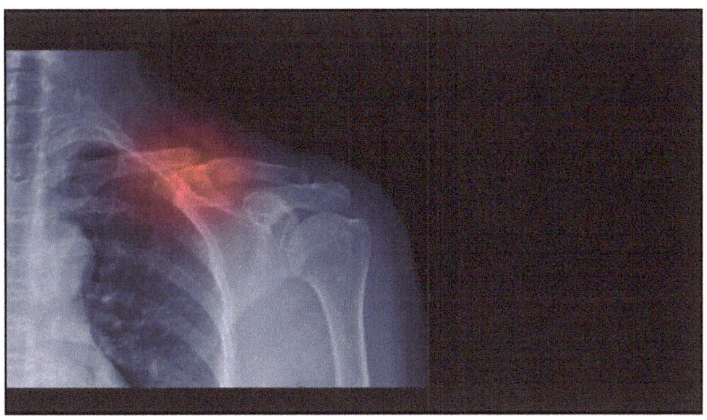

Acromioclavicular Joint Injury: **Seen after fall on shoulder**

Sx: Pain, swelling, bruising

PE:

Dx: AP X-ray

Tx:

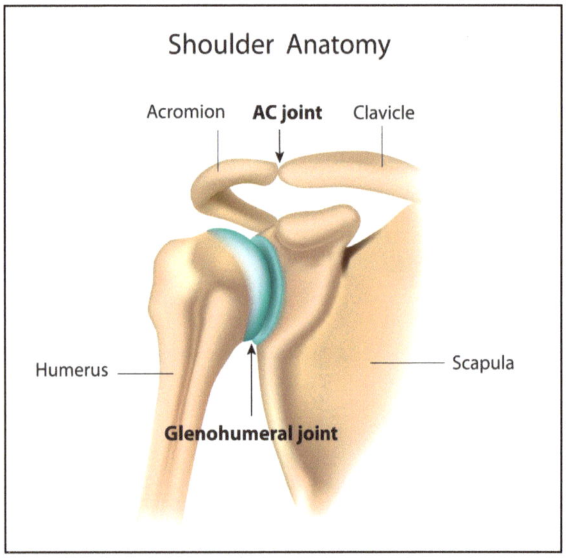

SLAP Lesion: **Labrum tear at bicep tendon attachment (anterior to posterior)**

Sx: Clicking, catching

PE:

Dx: O'Brien test

Tx:

Rotator Cuff Tendinopathy

Supraspinatus Tear:

Sx: Pain, weakness, diminished range of motion

PX:

Dx: (+) empty can, (+) arm drop

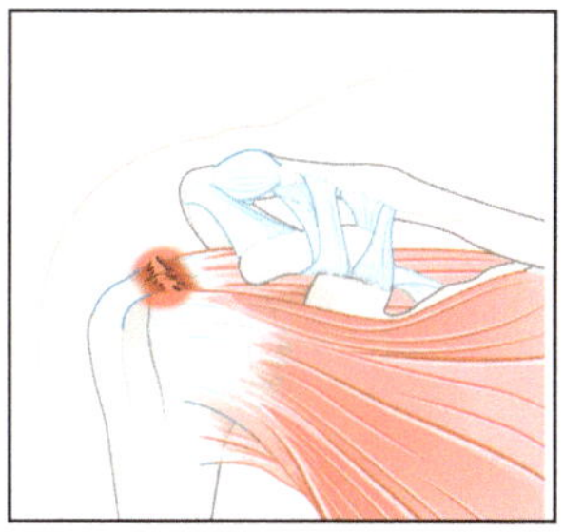

Tx:

Impingement Syndrome:

Sx: Pain, weakness, diminished range of motion

PE:

Dx: (+) Hawkin's, (+) Neer's

Tx:

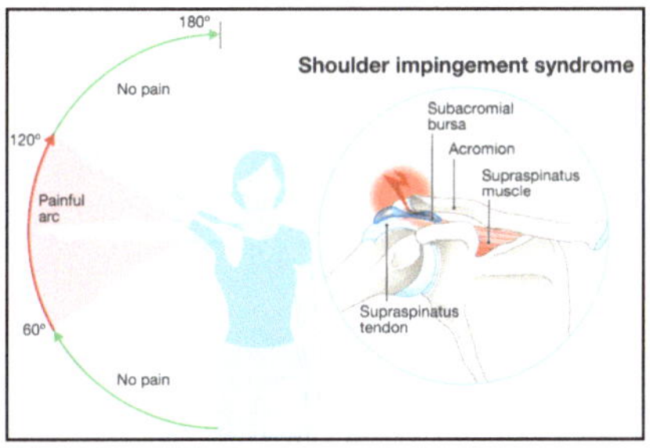

Thoracic Outlet Syndrome: **Compression of brachial plexus or subclavian vessels**

Sx: Pain in upper extremity, paresthesia's in lower extremities

PE:

Dx: (+) Adson's test, MRI, X-ray

Tx:

Subscapularis Tear: **Supraspinatus, infraspinatus, teres minor, subscapularis**

Sx: Pain, weakness, diminished range of motion

PE:

Dx: (+) lift off test

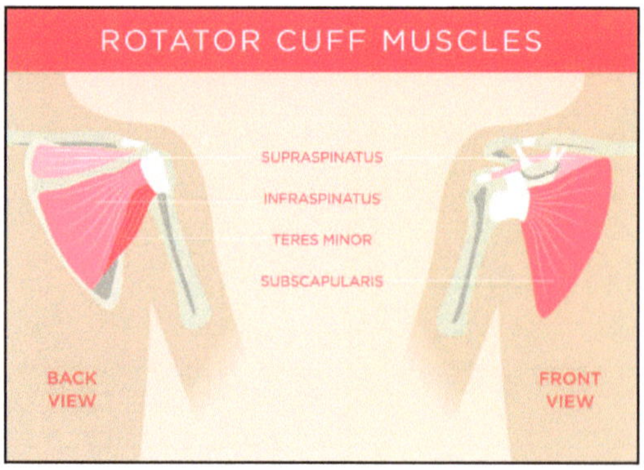

Tx:

Frozen Shoulder/Adhesive Capsulitis: **Inflammation/thickening - (common with diabetes)**

Sx: Decreased ROM (active & passive)

PE:

Dx: (+) Apley scratch

Tx:

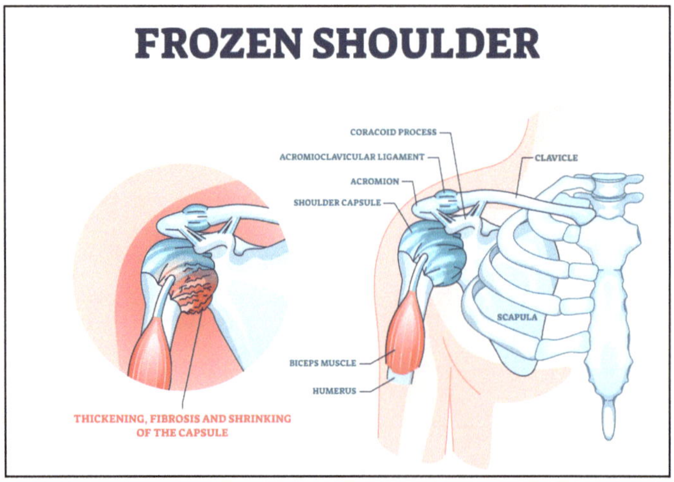

Disorders of the Knee

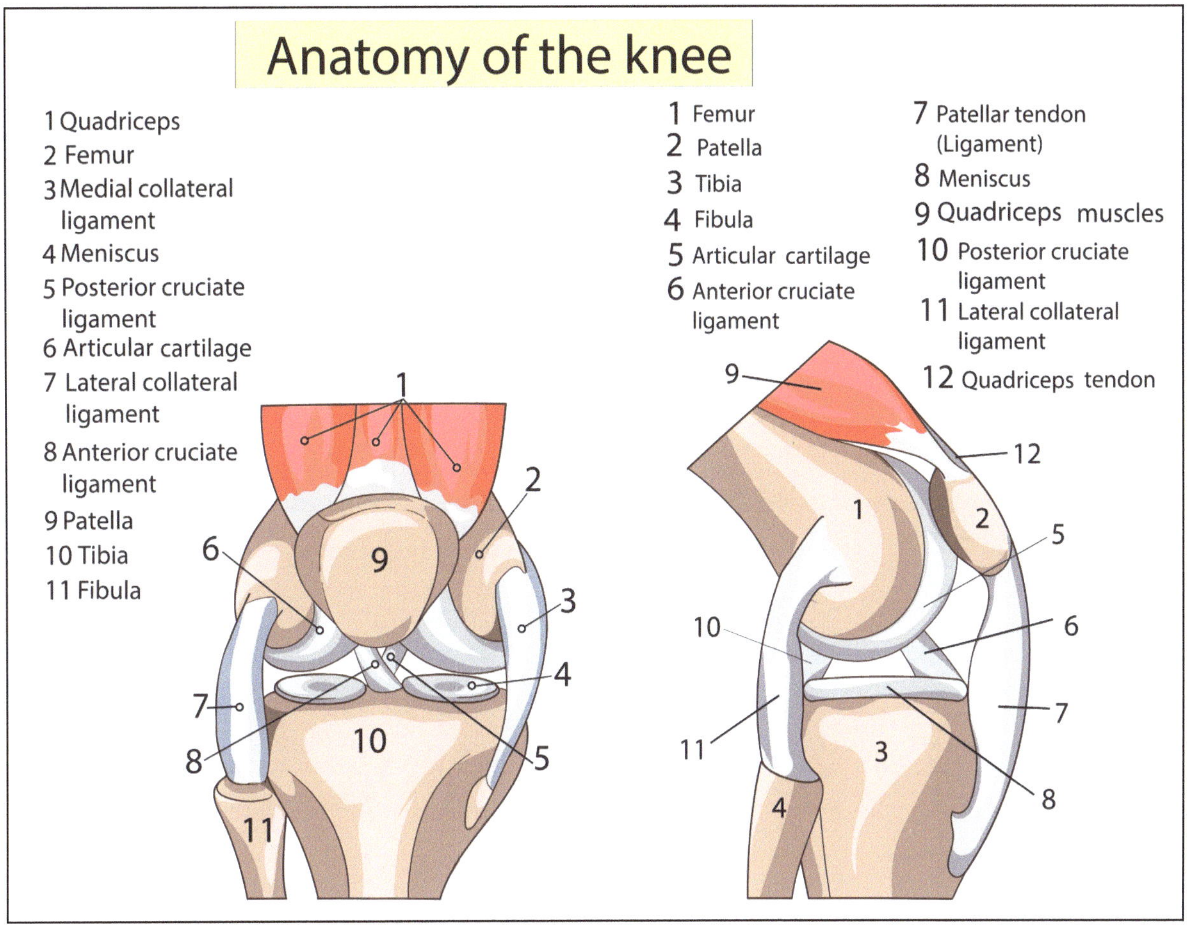

Patellofemoral Pain Syndrome: Softening of cartilage under patella with overuse

Risk Factors: Runners or cyclists, women

Sx: Anterior knee pain behind or around the patella worsened with knee hyperflexion

PE:

Dx: (+) Patellar grind, crepitus, positive apprehension sign

______________________________ **Tx:**

____

____

Ligament Injuries

Anterior Cruciate Ligament (ACL): **Most common pivoting injury, football & skiers**

Sx: "Pop", swelling & hemarthrosis, knee buckling, inability to bear weight

PE: (+) Lachmans (more specific than anterior drawer), pivot shift test

Dx: X-ray:

MRI:

___________________________________ Tx:

____

____

Posterior Cruciate Ligament (PCL): **Often with motor vehicle accidents**

Sx: Posterior knee pain, anterior bruising, large effusion

PE: (+) Posterior drawer

Dx:

___________________________________ Tx:

____

____

Medial Collateral Ligament (MCL) & Lateral Collateral Ligament (LCL):

Sx: Localized knee swelling, ecchymosis, stiffness

PE: MCL: Pain & laxity with (+) valgus stress

LCL: Pain & laxity with (+) varus stress

Dx:

___________________________________ Tx:

____

____

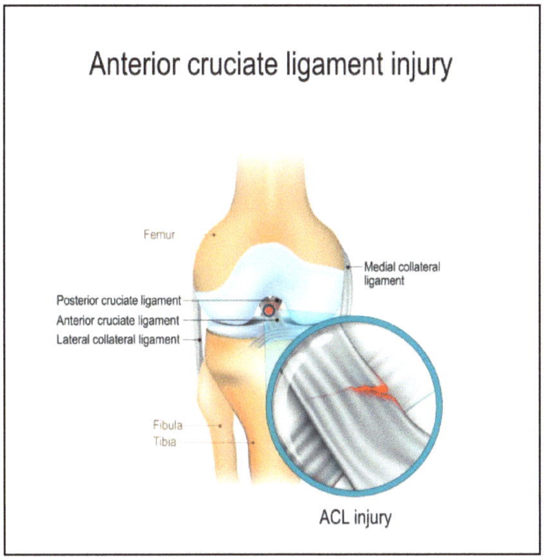

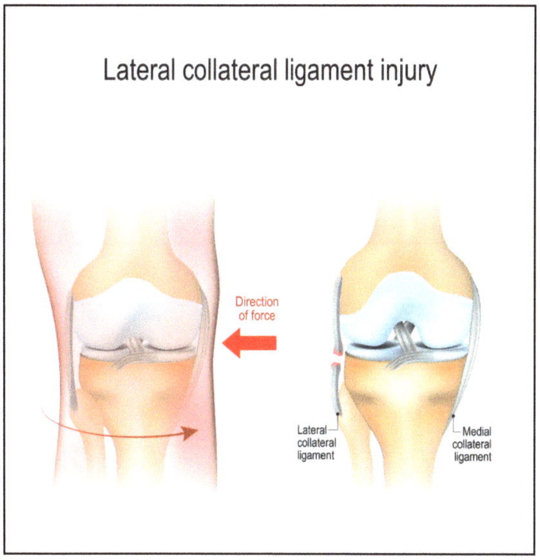

Meniscus Tear: **Twist injury - axial loading**

Sx: Popping & giving way, swelling after activities, joint effusion

PE: (+) McMurray's, (+) Apley compression

Dx:

______________________________ **Tx:**

____

____

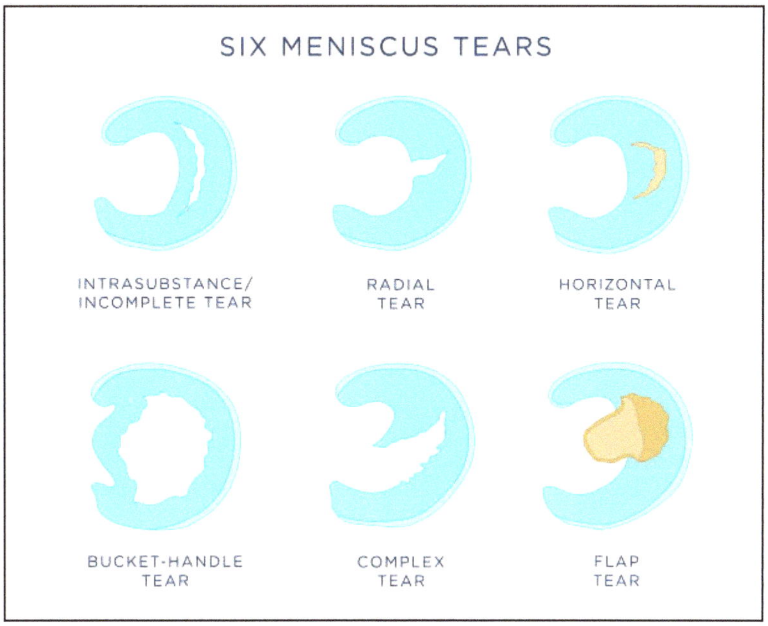

Patellar Tendonitis: **Activity related anterior knee pain, "jumper's knee"**

Sx: Tenderness inferior border of patella

PE: (+) Basset sign

Dx:

Tx:

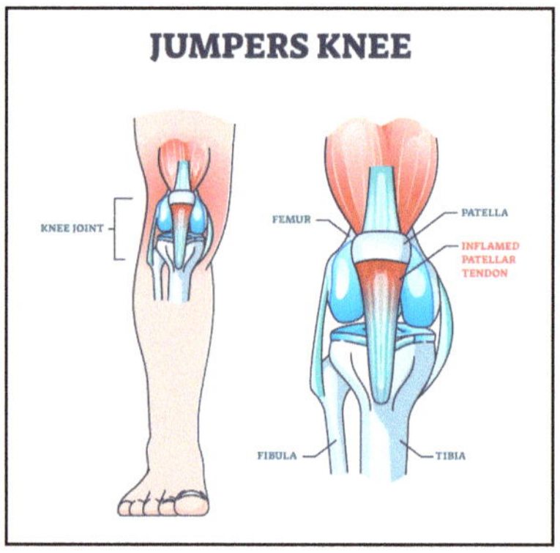

Patellar/Quad Tendon Rupture: **Fall on flexed knee**

Sx: Inability to extend knee, sharp knee pain with ambulation

- **Quadriceps:**
- **Patellar:**

PE:

Dx: X-ray (lateral view)

- **Quadriceps:**
- **Patellar:**

Tx:

Rupture of the quadriceps tendon

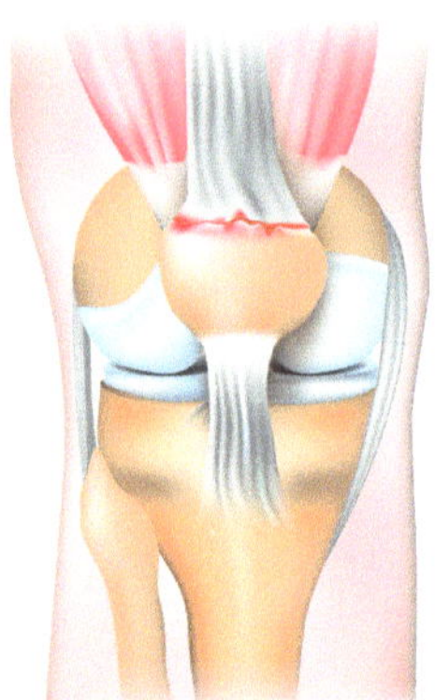

Patellar tendon rupture

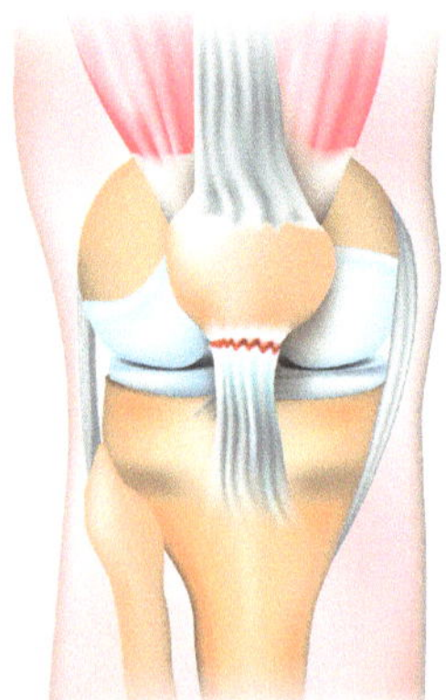

Patella Dislocation: Valgus stress after twisting injury - more common in women

Sx: Patella displaces laterally

PE:

Dx: X-ray

Tx:

Patella Fracture: Usually from direct blow

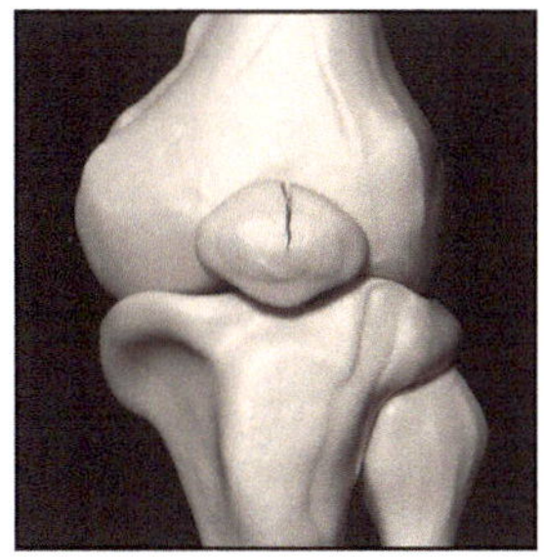

Sx: Pain, swelling, deformity, limited knee extension with pain

PE:

Dx: X-ray = sunrise view

Tx:

Baker's Cyst: Posterior knee cyst that contains synovial fluid

Sx: Bulge, knee pain, swelling

PE:

Dx: Doppler to rule out DVT and see fluid

Tx:

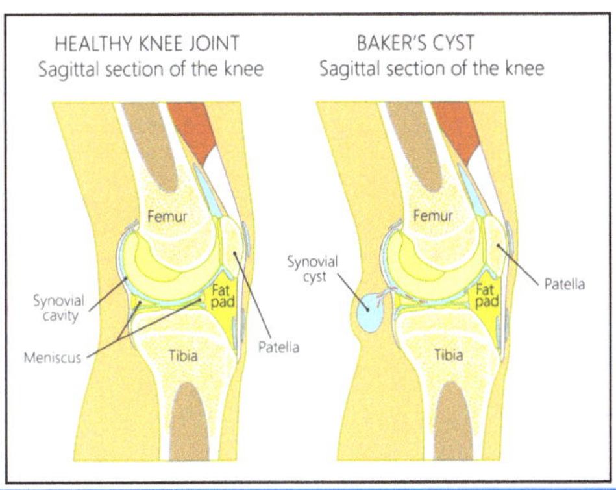

Tibial Plateau Fractures:

Sx:

PE: Knee effusion, pain

Dx: X-ray

Tx:

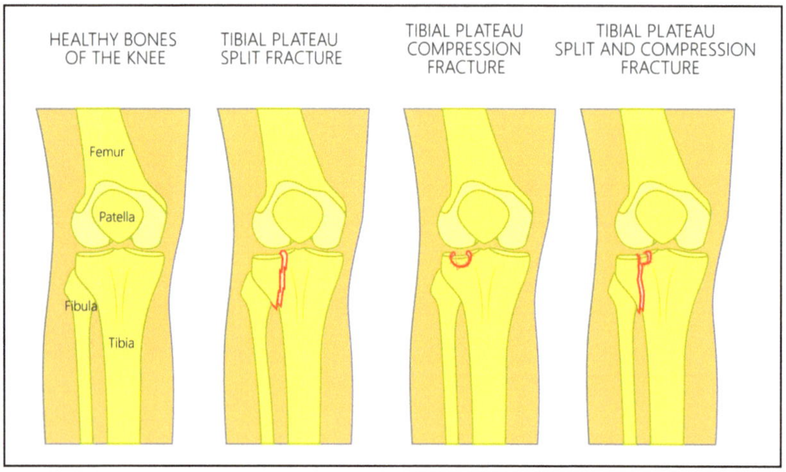

Femoral Condyle Fractures: Rare

Sx:

PE:

Dx: X-ray

Tx:

Disorders of the Ankle and Foot - *Splint & Ortho follow up*

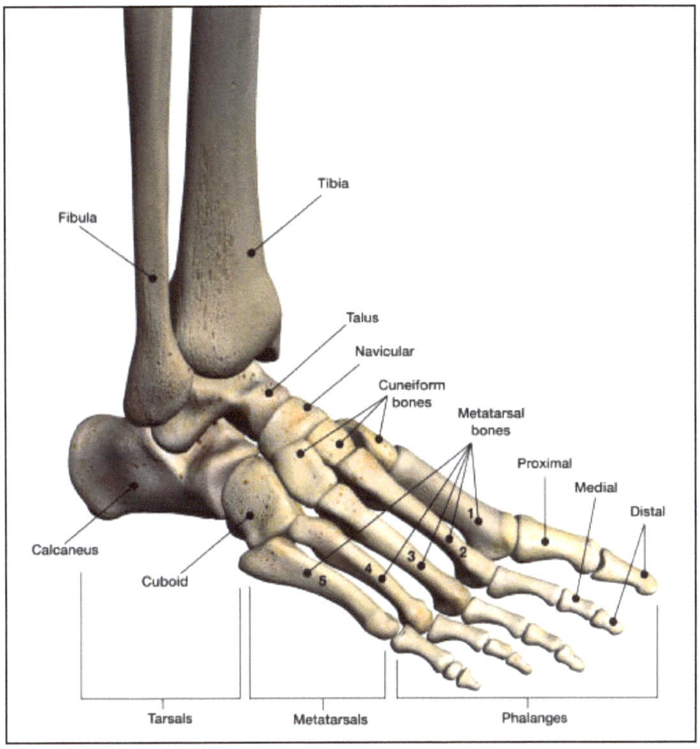

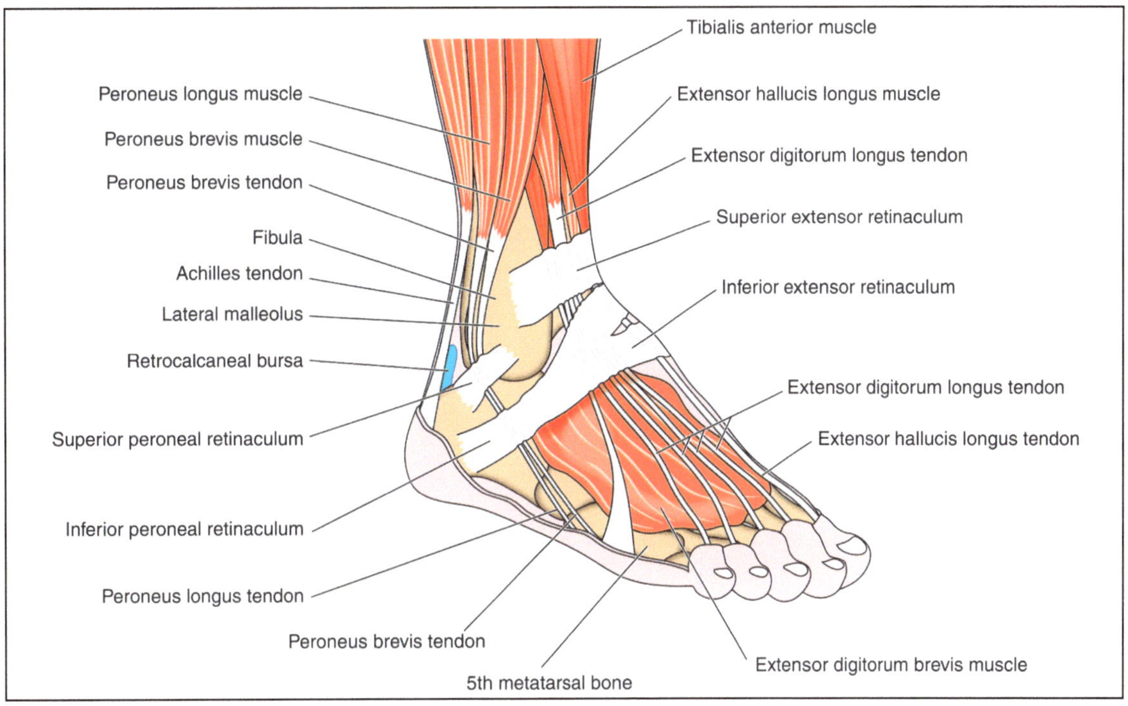

Ankle Sprain: **Most commonly the anterior talofibular ligament (ATFL)**

Sx: Grade 1:

Grade 2:

Grade 3:

Always look for Maisonneuve fracture then peroneal nerve involvement (foot drop and decreased sensation in digits 1 & 2)

PE: Anterior drawer

Talar tilt test

Dx:

______________________________ Tx:

____

____

Ankle Strain:

Sx: 1st degree: Minor tear of musculotendinous unit, swelling, local tenderness & minor loss of function

2nd degree: More fibers torn, but without complete disruption, greater swelling & ecchymosis, loss of strength

Dx:

______________________________ Tx:

____

____

Ottawa Ankle Rule

Syndesmotic Sprain:

Sx:

PX:

Dx: X-ray

___

___

___

Tx:

Achilles Tendon Rupture:

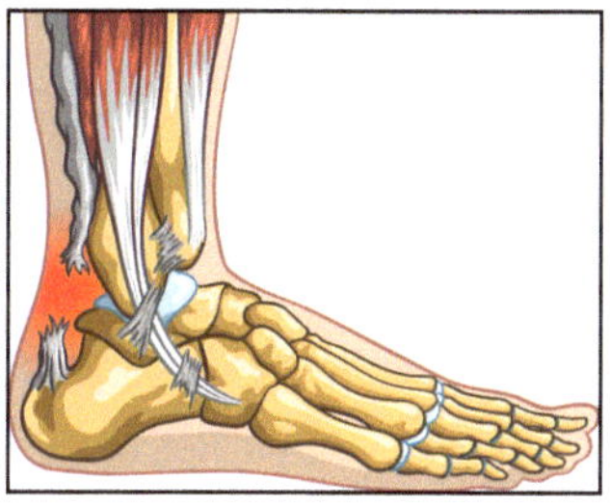

Risk Factors:

Sx: Inability to bear weight, "pop," sudden, sharp pain

PE: (+) Thompson

Dx:

___

___

___

Tx:

Bunion: Hallux valgus deformity leading to lateral deviation

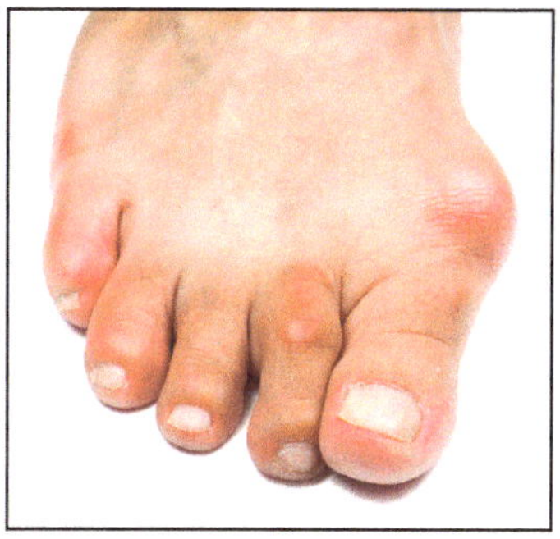

Risk Factors:

Sx: Pain over big toe at the MTP joint with lateral deformity

PE:

Dx:

___

___

___

Tx:

Jones Fracture: **Transverse fracture through the diaphysis of the 5th metatarsal**

***risk for non-union & re-fracture**

Sx: Pain over the fifth metatarsal with weight bearing

PE:

Dx: X-rays

______________________________ **Tx:**

____

____

Pseudo Jones: **Fracture of the proximal tuberosity of the 5th metatarsal**

Sx:

PE:

Dx: X-ray

______________________________ **Tx:**

____

____

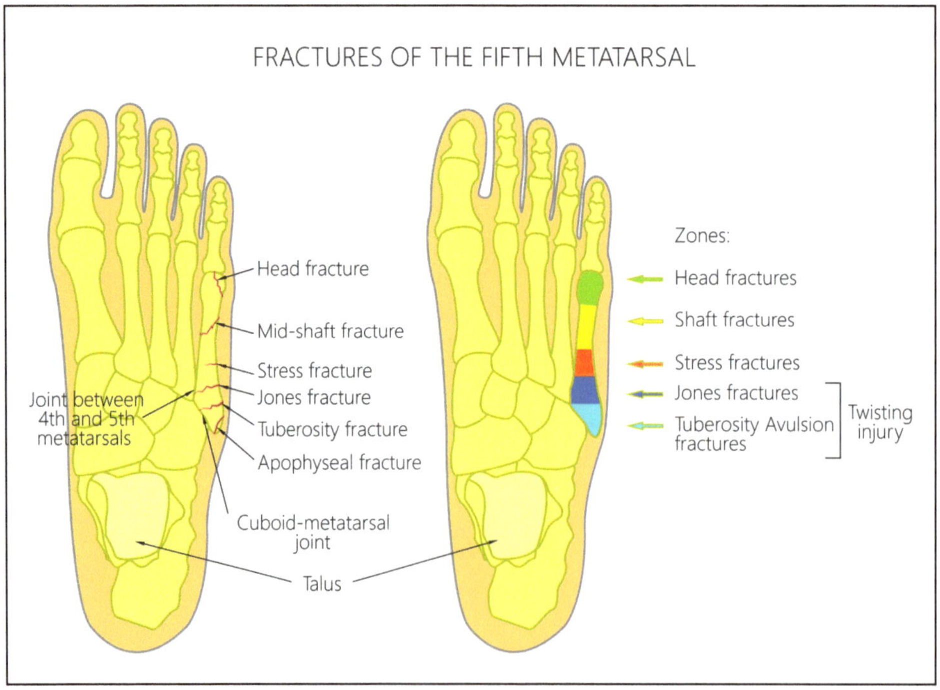

Lisfranc Injury: 1+ metatarsal bone displaces from tarsus

Sx: Severe pain, inability to bear weight

PE:

Dx: X-ray - fracture at the base of the 2nd metatarsal = pathognomonic

Tx:

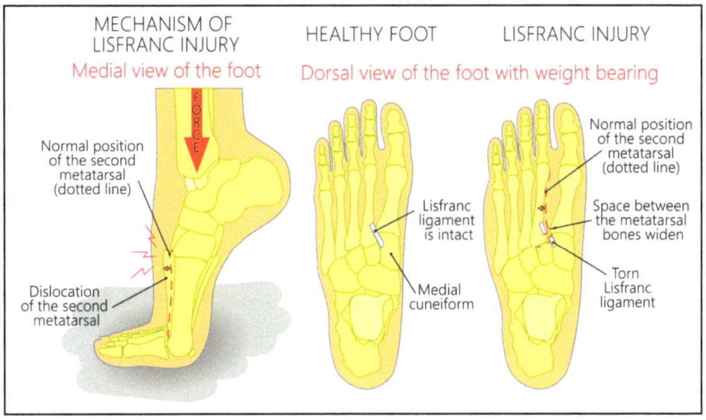

Plantar Fasciitis: Seen in athletes, one of the most common causes of foot pain in adults

Sx: Pain on plantar surface, inferior heel pain, usually worse after rest

PE: Local point tenderness, pain increases with dorsiflexion of toes

Dx:

Tx:

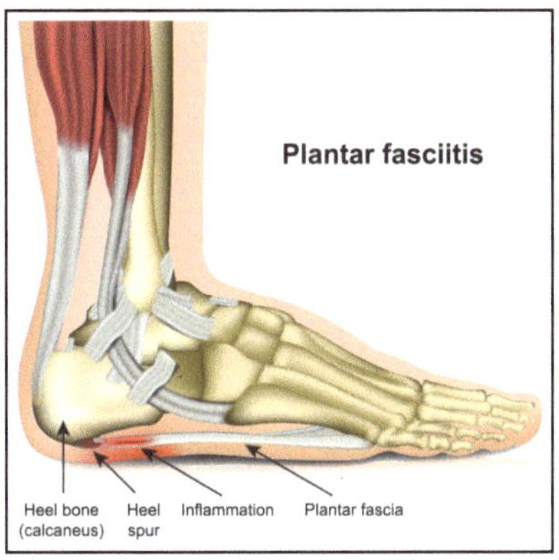

Morton's Neuroma: Painful mass near tarsal head

Sx: Sharp pain, possible numbness, burning pain, most common in the third intermetatarsal space

PE: Reproducible pain on palpation or squeezing the metatarsal Joints, clicking sensation "Mulder's sign"

Dx:

Tx:

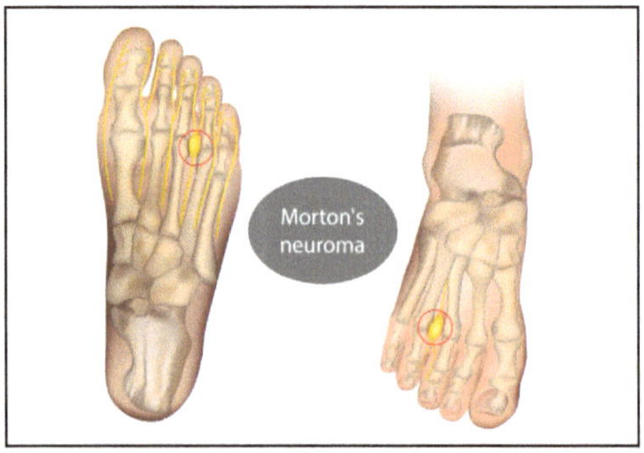

Tarsal Tunnel Syndrome: Posterior tibial nerve compression, travels through the tarsal tunnel

Sx: Pain increases throughout the day, worse at night, does not improve with rest

PE:

Dx:

Tx:

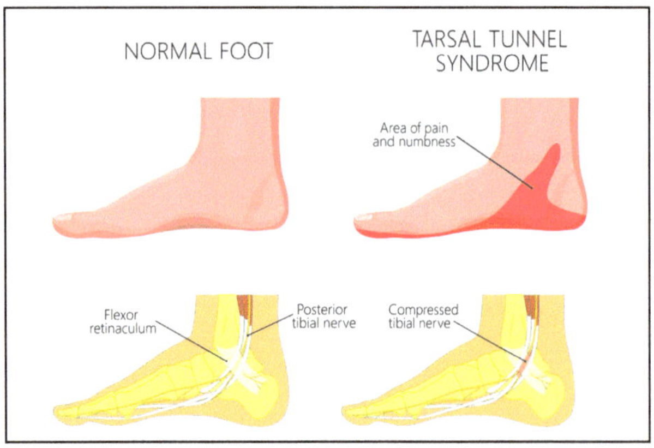

Pilon/Plafond Ankle Fracture: Distal tibia fracture from axial compression

Sx: Severe pain, swelling, deformity

PE:

Dx: X-ray

______________________________________ Tx:

____

____

Maisonneuve Fracture: Fracture or rupture of the deep deltoid ligament, usually from eversion ankle injury

*Proximal fibular fracture often in conjunction with:

1. Tearing of the distal talofibular syndesmosis and the interosseous membrane
2. Medial malleolus fracture

(Anyone with a distal ankle fracture should have proximal X-ray performed to rule out Maisonneuve fracture)

Sx:

PE:

Dx: X-ray

______________________________________ Tx:

____

____

Disorders of the Hip

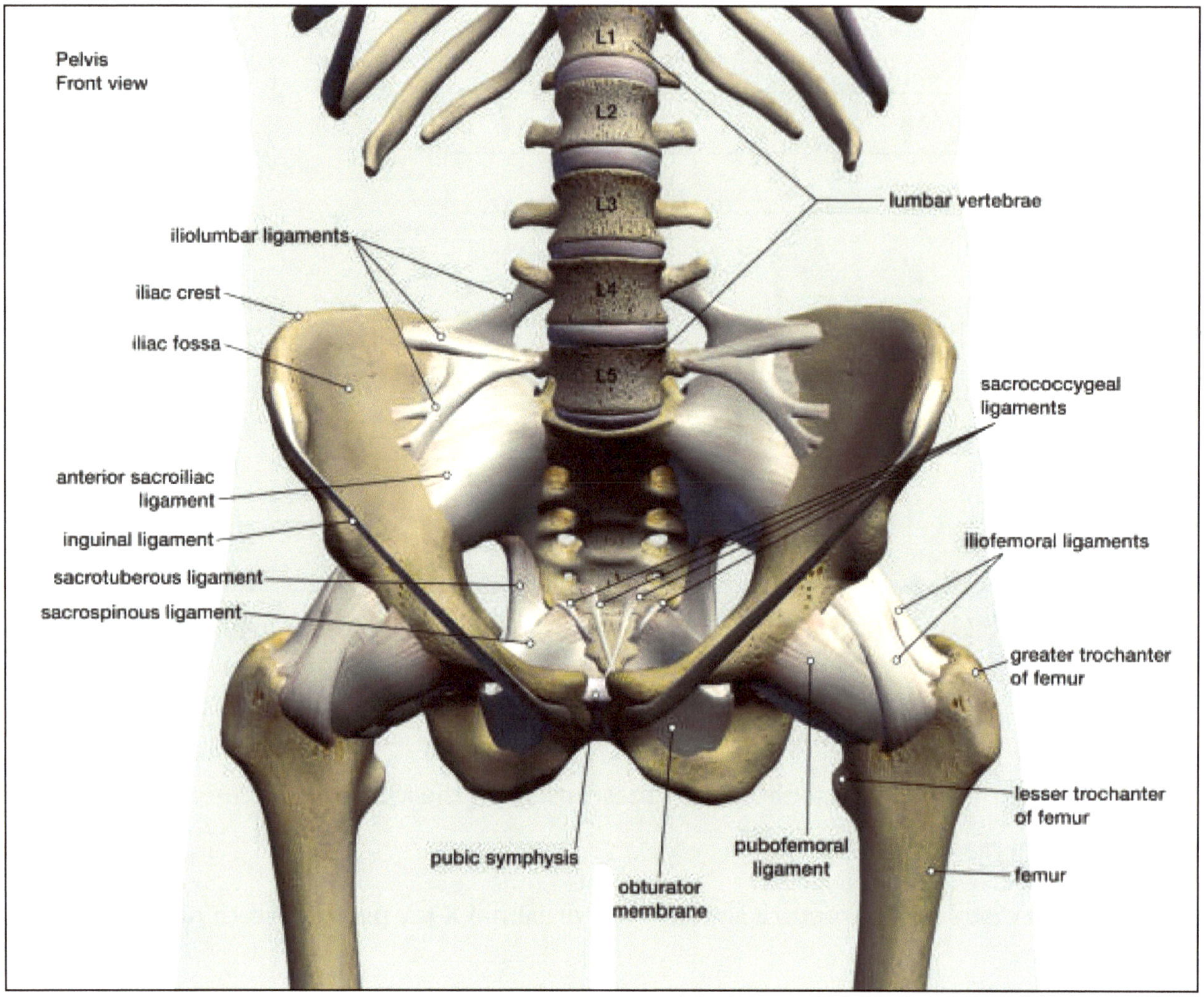

Avascular Necrosis of Hip (AVN): Insidious onset hip pain

Risk Factors:

Sx:

PE:

Dx: MRI

Tx:

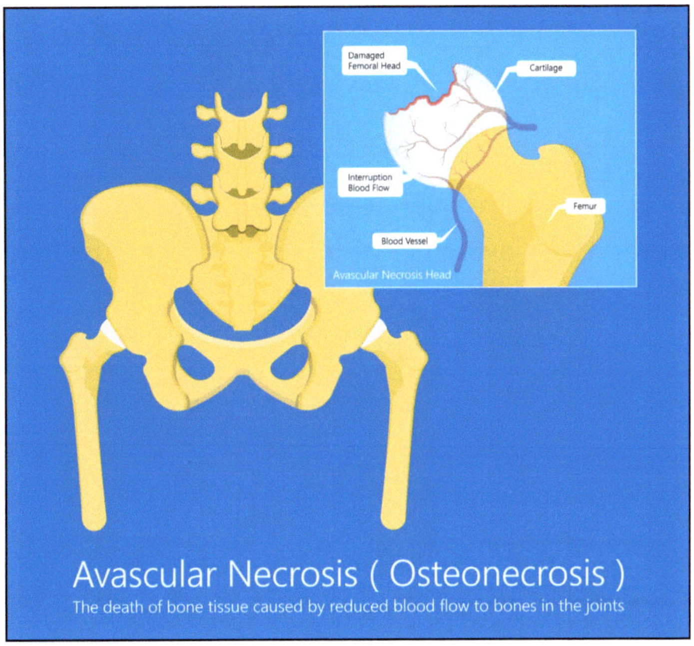

Legg-Calve-Perthes:

Risk Factors:

Sx: Hip pain, limp

PE:

Dx:

Tx:

Hip Dislocation:

Sx: Leg shortening, internal rotation & adduction, hip pain

Posterior:

Anterior:

PE:

Dx: X-ray, CT

Tx:

Hip Fracture: **Femoral head or neck fracture, risk of avascular necrosis most common in osteoporotic women**

Sx: Leg shortening, external rotation, abduction

PE:

Dx: X-ray

Tx:

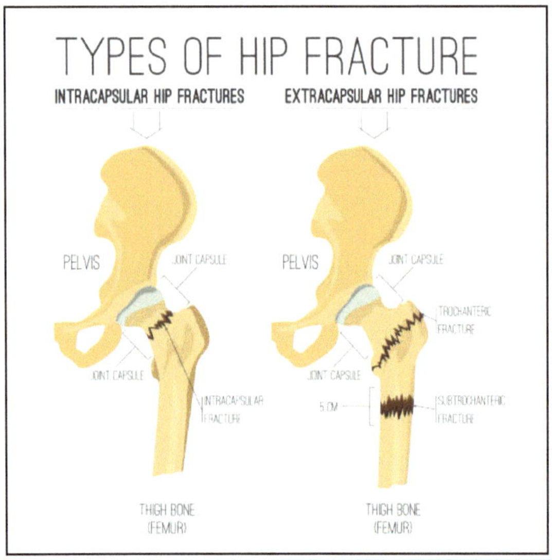

Pelvic Fractures: **High impact injuries i.e., motor vehicle injuries**

Sx: Pain with movement or inability to move

PE:

Dx: X-ray/CT scan

Tx:

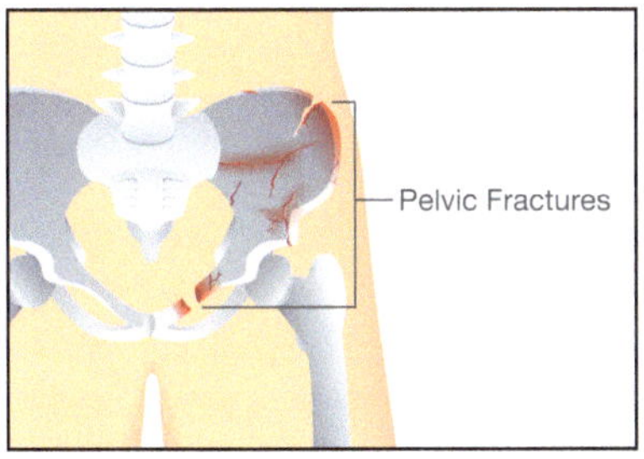

Iliotibial Band Syndrome: **Inflammation of the IT band**

Sx: Pain over lateral femoral epicondyle

PE:

Dx: Clinical, may see signs on US

Tx:

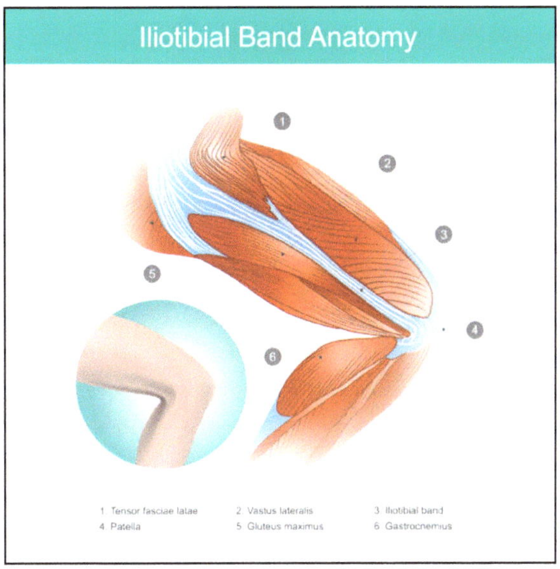

Spine Fractures

Clay Shoveler's Fracture:

Sx:

PE:

Dx: X-ray (lateral c-spine)

Tx:

Hangman's Fracture:

Sx: Pain

PE:

Dx: X-ray

Tx:

Jefferson Fracture: C1

Sx:

PE:

Dx: X-ray (odontoid and lateral c-spine), CT scan

Tx:

Odontoid Fracture: C2

Sx:

PE:

Dx: X-ray (odontoid view)

______________________________ Tx:

____

____

Basilar Skull Fracture:

Sx: Pain

PE:

Dx: X-ray

______________________________ Tx:

____

____

Atlanto-Axial Joint Dislocation:

Sx:

PE:

Dx: X-ray (odontoid view) or CT

______________________________ Tx:

____

____

Back Disorders

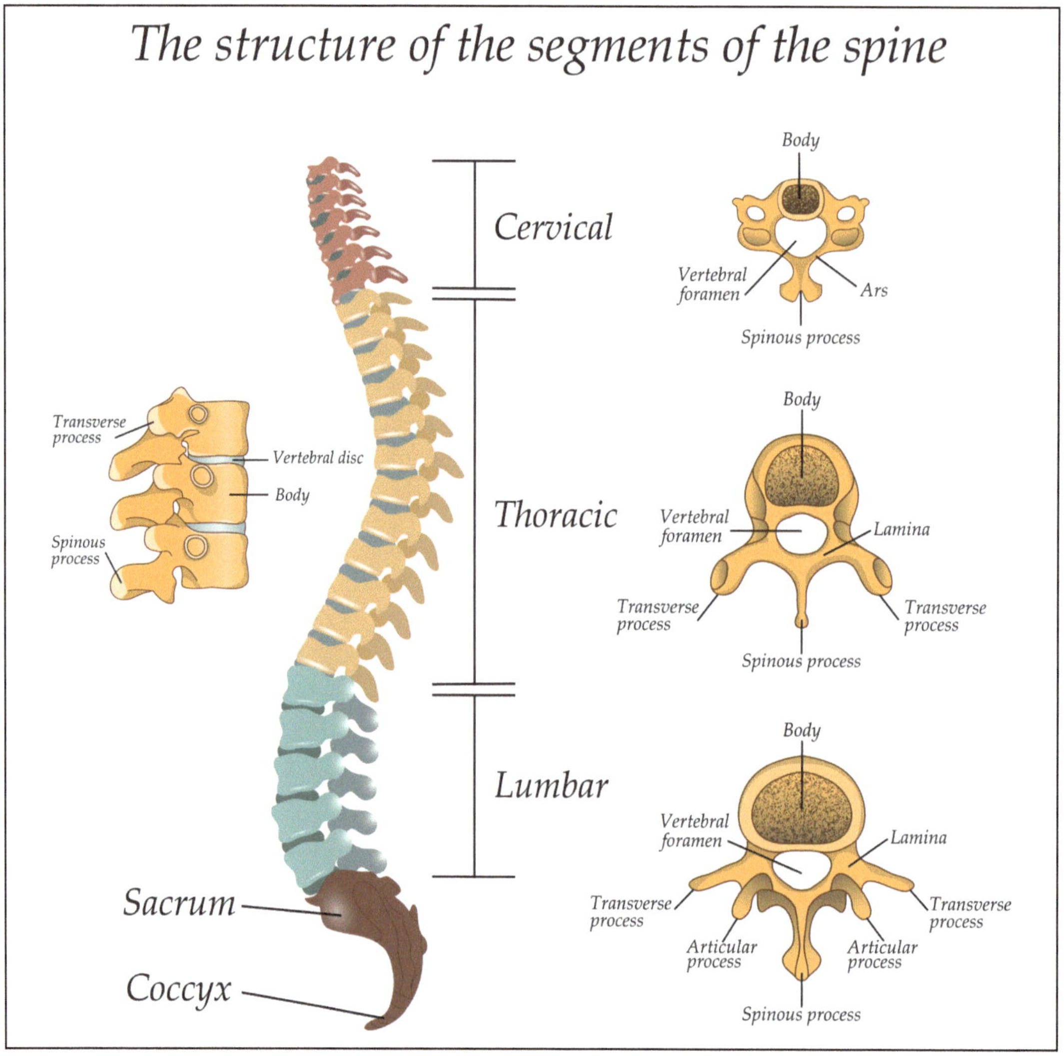

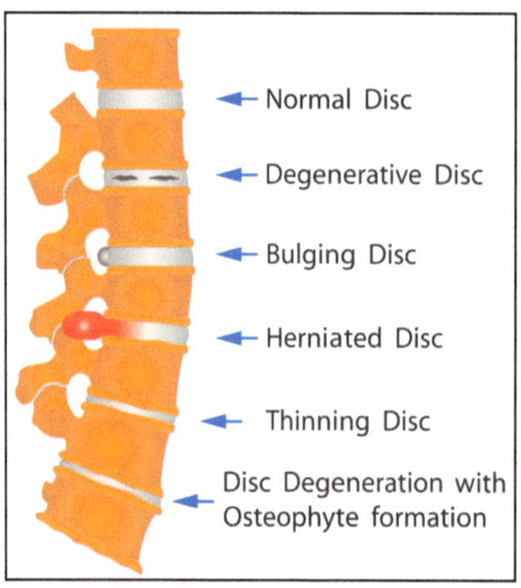

Ankylosing Spondylitis: **Seronegative spondyloarthropathy**

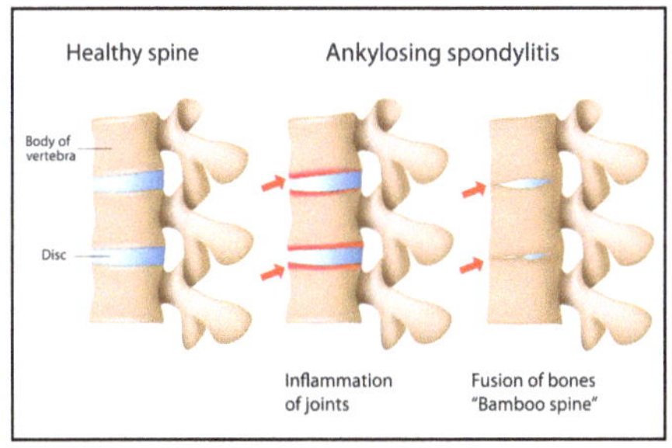

Sx: Back pain, stiffness, uveitis

PE:

Dx: (+) HLA-B27, bamboo spine

____

____

____

Tx:

Back Pain/Strain: **Back pain without neuro symptoms (radiculopathy)**

Sx: Pain

PE: (+) Palpation, (-) neuro exam, (-) straight leg raise, (-) Waddell's signs

Dx:

____

____

____

Tx:

Cauda Equina Syndrome: **Compression of nerve roots**

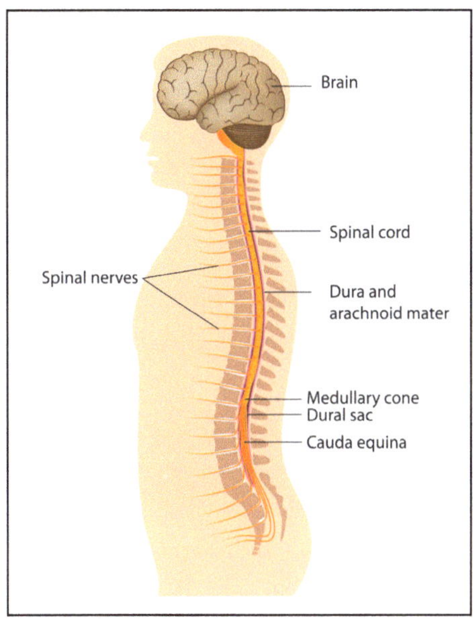

Sx: Saddle anesthesia, bladder/bowel incontinence

PE:

Dx: MRI

____

____

____

Tx:

Herniated Nucleus Pulposus: Causes nerve roots compression

C-Spine:

Sx:

Tx:

PE: (+) Spurling test

Dx:

Lumbosacral Spine:

Sx:

Tx:

PE: (+) Straight leg raise

Dx:

Spinal Stenosis: Narrowing leads to compression of nerve roots

Sx: "Shopping cart sign"

PE:

Dx: (+) Kemp sign - pain with extension

Tx:

spinal stenosis

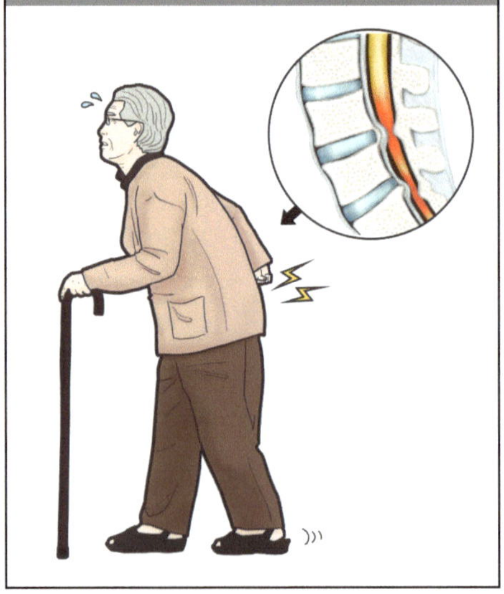

Kyphosis:

Sx:

PE: Abnormal curving of the T-spine (upper back)

Dx:

Spondylosis: **Osteoarthritis of the spine**

Sx: Limitations of lumbar flexibility & tight hamstring

PE:

Dx: X-ray, MRI

Tx:

Spondylolysis: **Stress fracture through pars interarticularis defect**

Sx: Limitations of lumbar flexibility & tight hamstring

PE:

Dx: X-ray, MRI

Tx:

Spondylolisthesis: **Slipping of vertebrae (worsening of spondyloysis)**

Sx: Pain when it progresses

PE:

Dx: X-ray = "Scottie dog"

Tx:

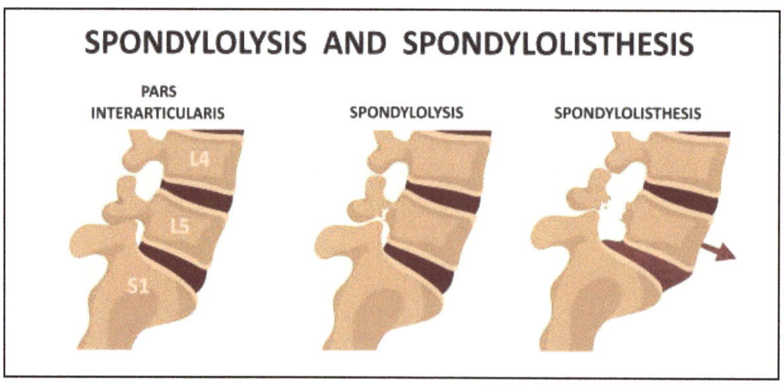

Spinal Epidural Abscess: Most common pathogen is S. aureus

Sx:

PE:

Dx: Spinal MRI

Tx:

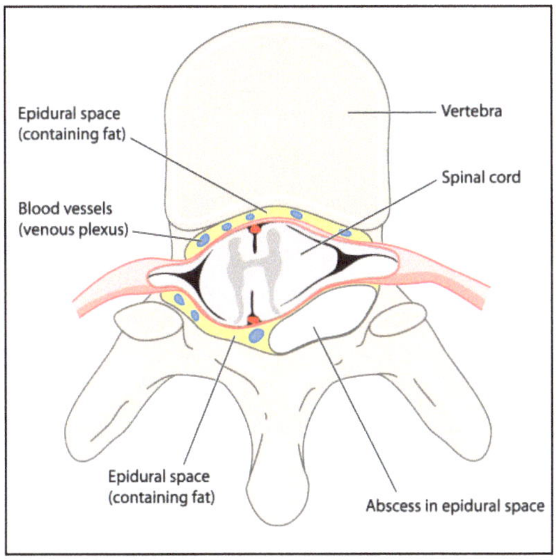

Scoliosis:

Sx:

PE: Adams forward bend test, scoliometer

Dx: X-ray

Tx:

Other MSK Disorders

Compartment Syndrome: Muscle & nerve ischemia

Sx:

PE: 6Ps - pain, pallor, pulselessness, paralysis, pokilothermia, paresthesia's

Dx: Pressure > 30-45 mmHg

Tx:

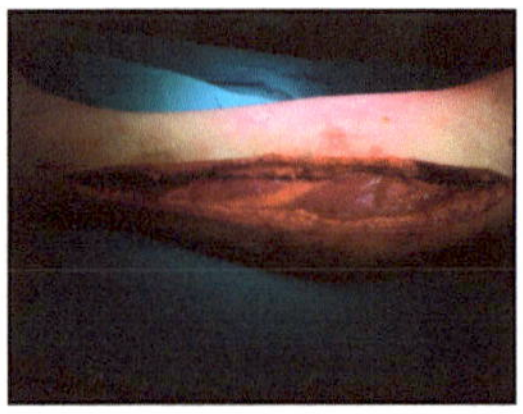

Osteoarthritis: Wear and tear

Sx: Morning stiffness, stiffness worse with use, better with rest

PE: Bouchard (PIP) vs Heberden nodes (DIP)

Dx: X-ray:

Tx:

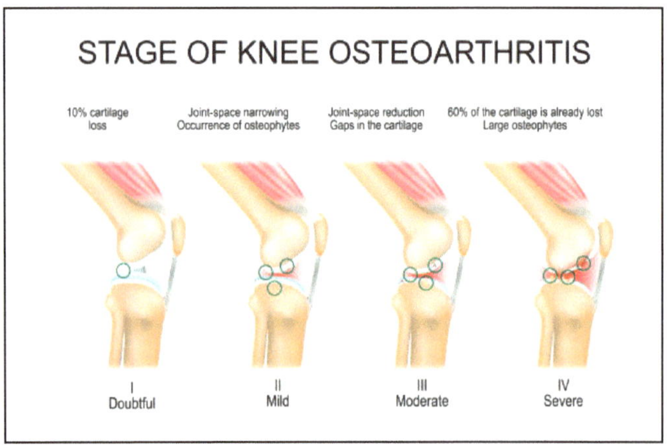

Osteoporosis: **Thinning of bony trabeculae**

Risk Factors:

Sx:

PE:

Dx: DEXA with BMD < -2.5

Tx:

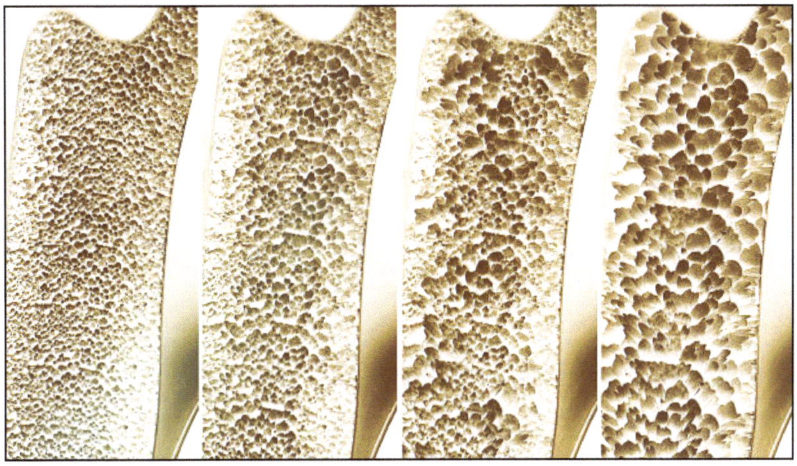

Ganglion Cyst:

Sx: Tender or non-tender dorsal wrist mass

PE:

Dx: Transillumination

Tx:

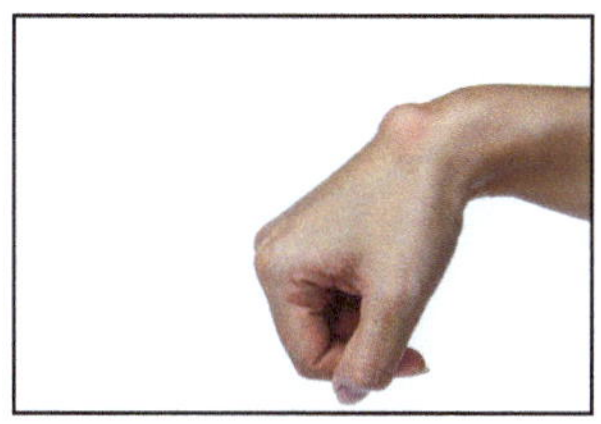

Rhabdomyolysis: Breakdown & necrosis of skeletal muscle

Risk Factors:

Sx: Muscle pain & weakness, tea colored urine

PE:

Dx: CK, urinalysis, CBC, CMP, ECG

Tx:

Paget's Disease: Of bone

Sx: Asymptomatic, bone deformity, pathologic fracture, arthritis, pain

PE:

Dx:

Pectus Excavatum:

Sx: Sternal depression

PE:

Dx: Clinical, can do CT if severe

Pectus Carinatum:

Sx: Protrusion of sternum

PE:

Dx: Clinical, X-ray

Bone Tumors

Osteosarcoma: **Malignant bone tumor seen in kids and adults > 65**

Rare form of cancer

Most common form of cancer in patients < 20 years of age

Sx: Pain worse at night, localized bone pain

PE:

Dx: X-ray: "sunburst", "hair on ends", Codman's Triangle

Biopsy:

Tx:

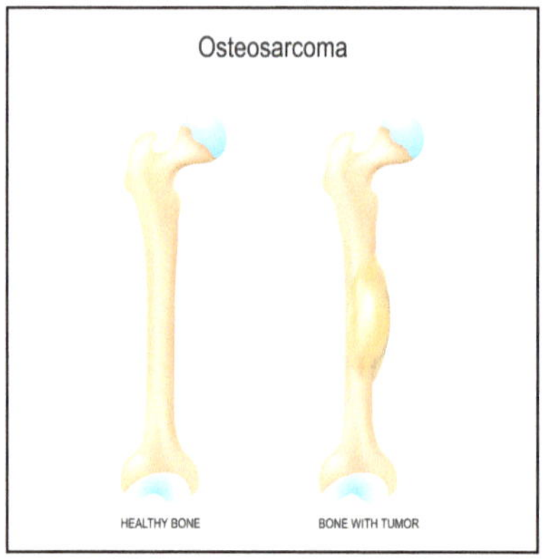

Ewing Sarcoma: **Malignant bone tumor, most common in femur and pelvis of kids**

Sx: Fever, bone pain, possibly systemic systems

PE:

Dx: X-ray: "onion skin" and/or "moth-eaten" appearance, Codman's Triangle

Labs:

Tx:

Chondrosarcoma: **Primary malignant cartilage cancer**

Sx: Constant, deep, achy pain especially @ night, *not relieved by rest*

PE:

Dx: X-ray:

CT or MRI:

Tx:

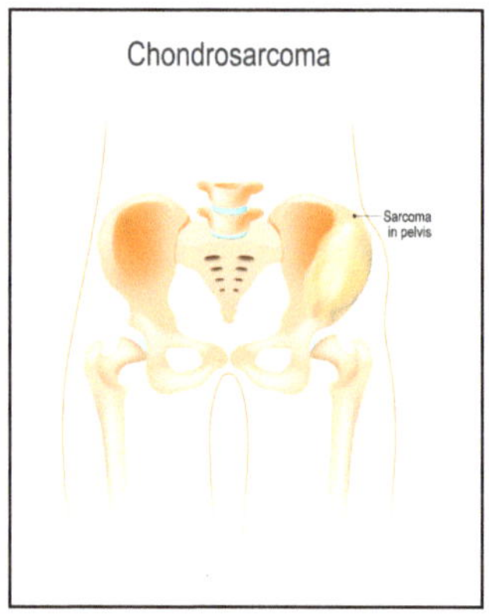

Osteochondroma: **Benign bone tumor, most common in male kids 10-20 years old**

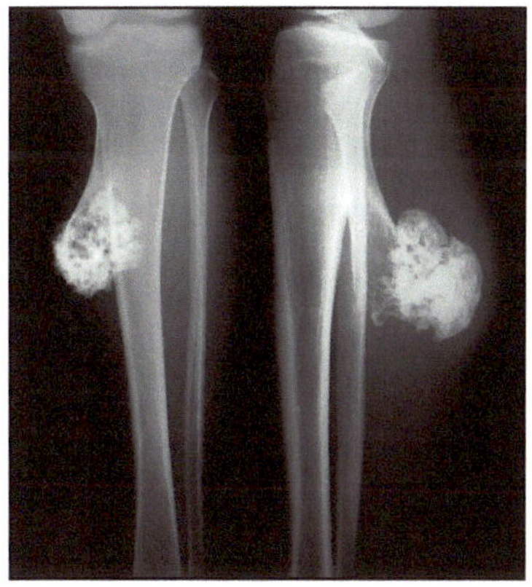

Sx:

PE:

Dx: X-ray: pedunculated lesion in the medullary cavity

Biopsy:

Tx:

Fibrosarcoma: **Lytic lesions**

Sx: Painless/tender mass, pain

PE:

Dx: X-ray, MRI, CT, biopsy

Tx:

Osteoid Osteoma: **Benign tumor in children 5-20 years old**

Sx: Increased pain @ night unrelated to activity, relieved by aspirin

PE:

Dx: X-ray: small radiolucent nidus (produces high levels prostaglandins)

CT/MRI:

Tx:

Infectious MSK Disorders

Osteomyelitis: Infection of the bone & marrow
Most common in femur & tibia = children
Most common in vertebrae = adults

Sx: Fever, chills, bone pain, decreased range of motion, difficulty bearing weight

PE:

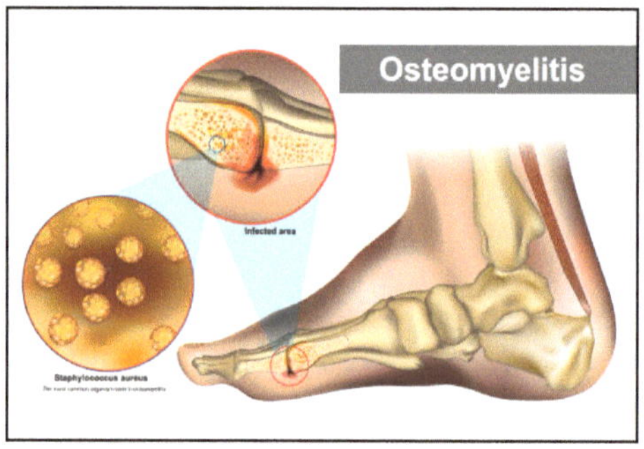

Dx: Labs: increased CRP & ESR, possibly WBC
X-ray:
MRI:
Bone aspiration:

Tx:

Septic Arthritis: Bacteria in the joint cavity
Medical emergency - can rapidly destroy joints

Knee:
Hip:
Sternoclavicular joint:

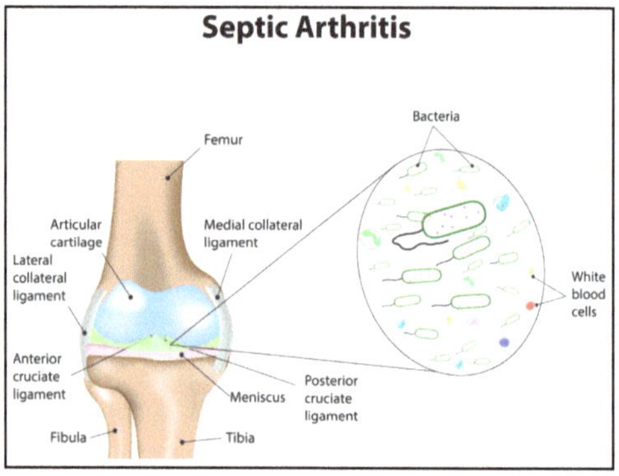

Sx: Swollen, warm, painful and tender joint

PE:

Dx:
Labs:
Arthrocentesis with WBC > 25,000:
MRI/CT:

Tx:

Synovial Fluid Analysis:

Rheumatologic MSK Disorders

Fibromyalgia: Widespread muscular pain

Sx: Chronic, extreme fatigue, "fibro fog", neuro symptoms, headache

PE:

Dx: Clinical diagnosis of exclusion, need 11 of 18 trigger points, normal labs

____

____

____

Tx:

Sjögren's Syndrome: Autoimmune vs exocrine glands (salivary & lacrimal glands)

Sx: Dry mouth, dry eyes, vaginal dryness, bilateral parotid gland enlargement, dental caries

PE:

Dx: (+) Anti-Ro (SSA), (+) Anti-La (SSB), (+) RF, Schirmer's test < 5mm

____

____

____

Tx:

Systemic Lupus Erythematosus (SLE): Multi-organ autoimmune disorder of connective tissue

Sx: Malar rash, joint pain, renal, fever, pulmonary, night sweats

Systemic:

Discoid Lupus:

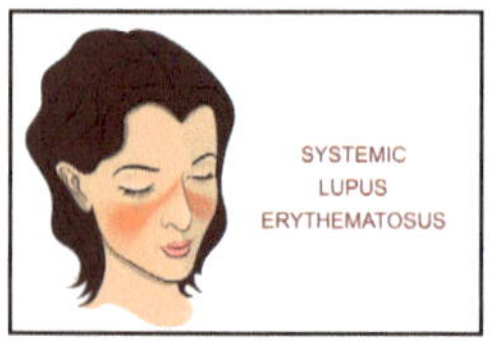

PE:

Dx: (+) ANA, (+) anti-dsDNA & (+) anti-smith (pathognomonic & specific for SLE), antiphospholipid antibodies

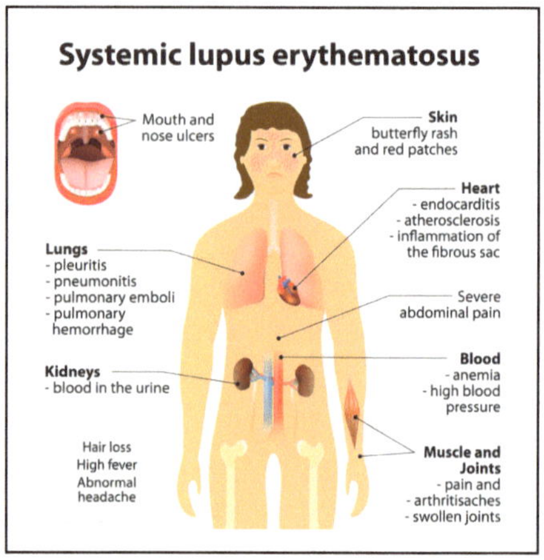

Tx:

**Drug Induced Lupus:*

Antiphospholipid Syndrome:

Sx: Recurrent DVT's or pulmonary embolisms, livedo reticularis

Recurrent miscarriages, valvular heart disease, neuro symptoms (stroke, TIA)

PE:

Dx: Labs: anticardiolipin antibodies, lupus anticoagulant (increased PTT)

Tx:

Scleroderma: Autoimmune connective tissue disorder - EXCESS Collagen

Sx: Shiny, thickened skin & tightness, interstitial lung disease, hypertension, esophageal hypomotility

CREST:

PE:

Dx: (+) ANA, (+) anti-centromere ab, (+) anti-SCL-70 ab

____

____

____

Tx: Specific to organ

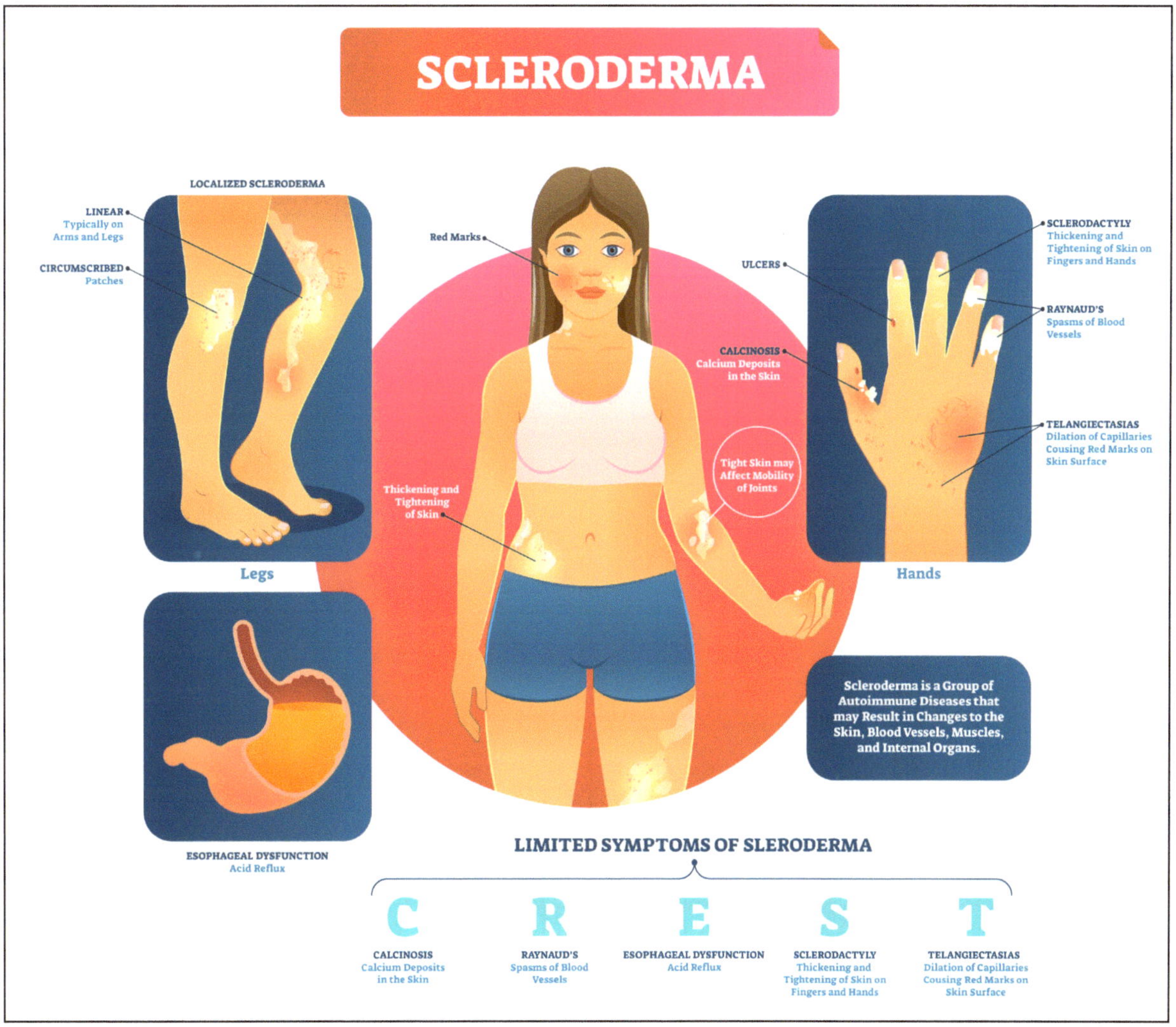

Polyarteritis Nodosa: **Small & medium vessel vasculitis of many organs**

Sx: Joint & muscle pain, Rosary sign

PE: Livedo reticularis & palpable purpura

Dx:

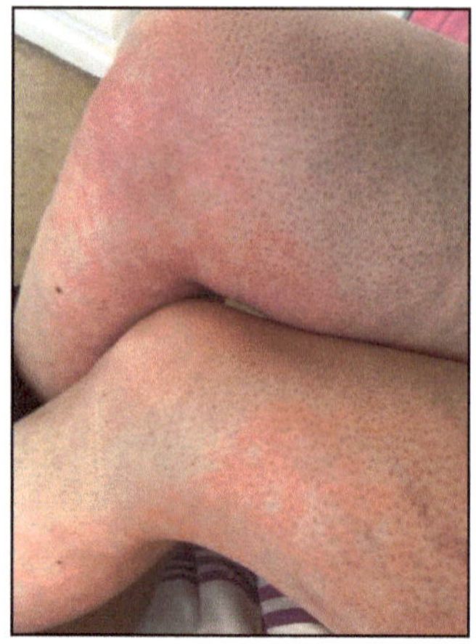

Tx:

Rheumatoid Arthritis: **Autoimmune inflammatory disorder with symmetric polyarthritis**

Sx:

PE: Morning stiffness > 1 hour - improves later in the day

Inflamed, small joints including MCP, PIP, MTP

Dx: Labs:

X-ray:

Tx:

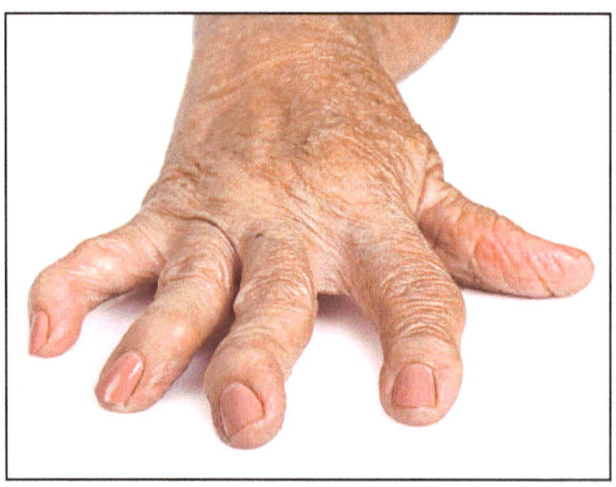

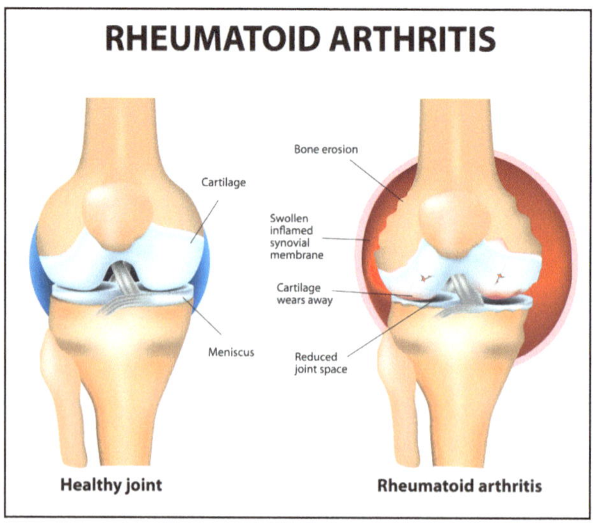

Polymyositis: Idiopathic autoimmune disorder leads to inflammatory muscle disease

Sx: Progressive symmetric proximal muscle weakness (shoulders, hips)

PE:

Dx: Labs:

Muscle or skin biopsy:

Tx:

Dermatomyositis: Polymyositis + skin involvement

Sx:

PE:

Dx: Labs:

Muscle Biopsy:

Tx:

Dermatomyositis

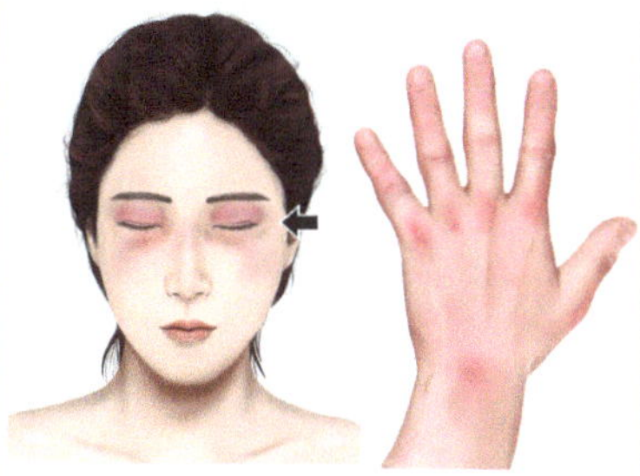

Polymyalgia Rheumatica (PRM): Inflammatory joint disease, idiopathic

Sx: Painful synovitis, bursitis, tenosynovitis, proximal joints, worse in AM - better with movement, *associated with Giant Cell Arteritis*

PE:

Dx:

Tx:

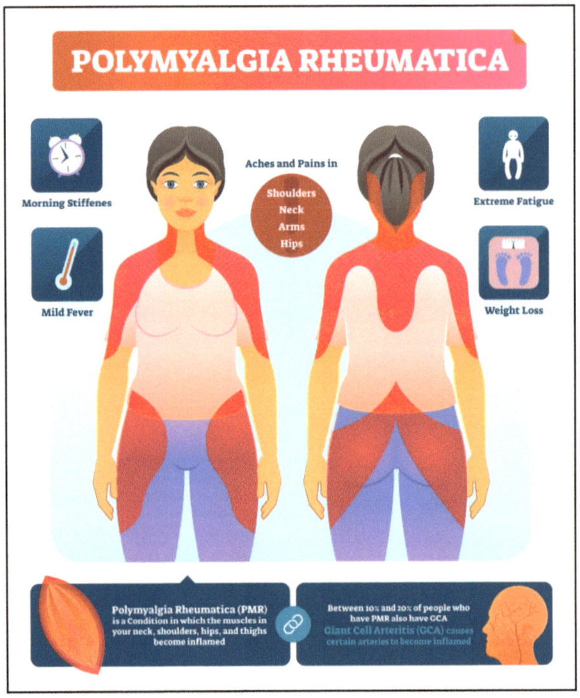

Reactive Arteritis (Reiter's): Autoimmune response to another infection most commonly after chlamydia or shigella

Sx: Can't see, pee or climb tree -- conjunctivitis, uveitis, urethritis, arthritis - ASYMMETRIC

PE:

Dx: +HLA-B27

Tx:

Juvenile Idiopathic Arthritis: Rheumatoid arthritis prior to age 16

Still's disease:

Sx: Fevers, body aches, rash, hepatosplenomegaly

PE:

Dx: Labs:

______________________________ **Tx:**

____

____

Psoriatic Arthritis: Seronegative spondylarthritis

Sx: Dactylitis, swollen fingers, silver scaly lesions

PE:

Dx: Labs:

X-ray:

______________________________ **Tx:**

____

____

SERONEGATIVE SPONDYLOARTHRITIS = REACTIVE ARTERITIS, PSORIATIC ARTHRITIS, IBD, ANKYLOSING SPONDYLITIS

Other Rheumatologic Conditions

Gout: Monosodium urate crystals

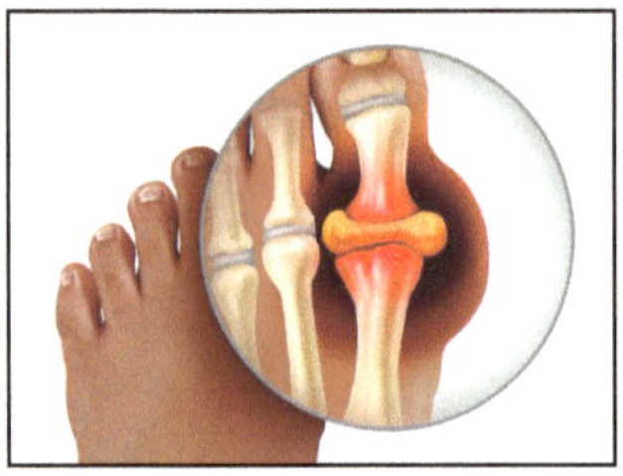

Risk Factors:

Sx: Rapid onset severe pain, joint stiffness, tenderness, tophi

PE:

Dx: Needle-shaped crystals + negative birefringence

Tx:

Pseudogout: Calcium pyrophosphate dihydrate

Sx: Painful, tender joint

PE:

Dx:

Tx:

Takayasu Arteritis: Large-vessel vasculitis

Sx: Syncope, chest pain, asymmetric BP in arms

PE:

Dx: Angiography with stenosis, bruit of aorta

Tx:

Kawasaki Syndrome: **Vasculitis seen in young children**

Sx: CRASH and burn (conjunctivitis, rash, adenopathy, strawberry tongue, hand-foot edema, fever > 3 days)

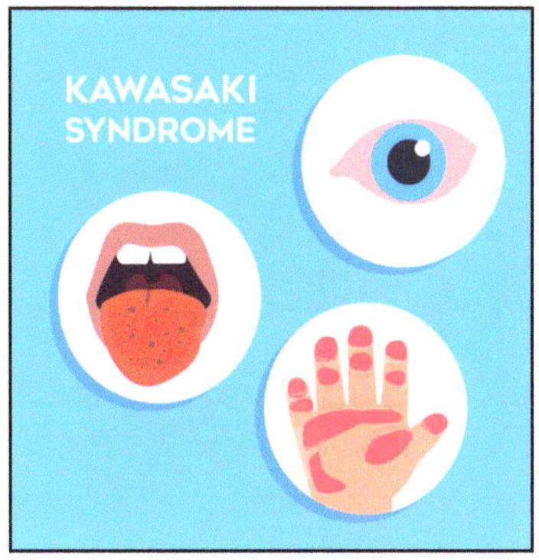

PE:

Dx: ECHO w/ coronary artery aneurysms, high ESR & CRP

____

____

____

Tx:

Granulomatosis W/Polyangiitis (Wegener's): **Vasculitis**

Sx: Saddle nose, chronic rhinitis, glomerulonephritis, uveitis, hoarse voice

PE:

Dx: cANCA, biopsy with granulomas

____

____

____

Tx:

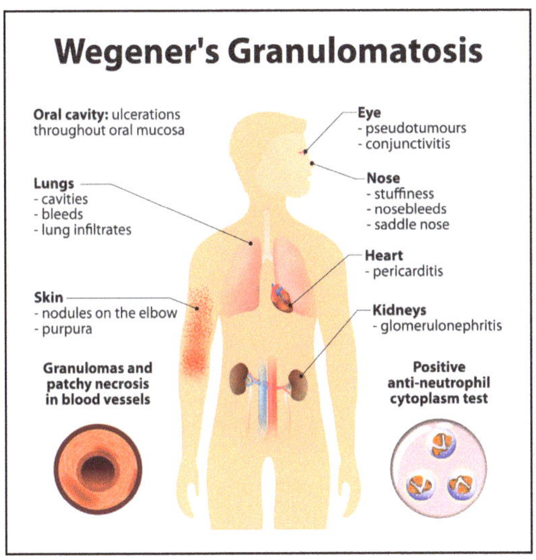

Eosinophilic Granulomatosis W/Polyangiitis (Churg-Strauss): Small & med vessel vasculitis, lung & renal involvement

Sx: Chronic sinusitis, asthma, blood eosinophilia

PE:

Dx: pANCA, high IgE, biopsy, ECG, ECHO

Tx:

Microscopic Polyangiitis: Small vessel vasculitis

Sx: Hypertension, nephritis, pulmonary hemorrhage, purpura (no nasopharynx symptoms)

PE:

Dx: Biopsy without granulomas, increased pANCA

Tx:

IgA Vasculitis (Henoch-Schönlein Purpura): Small vessel vasculitis (seen in young children after URI)

Sx: Purpura of lower extremities, nephritis

PE:

Dx: High IgA, no ANCA

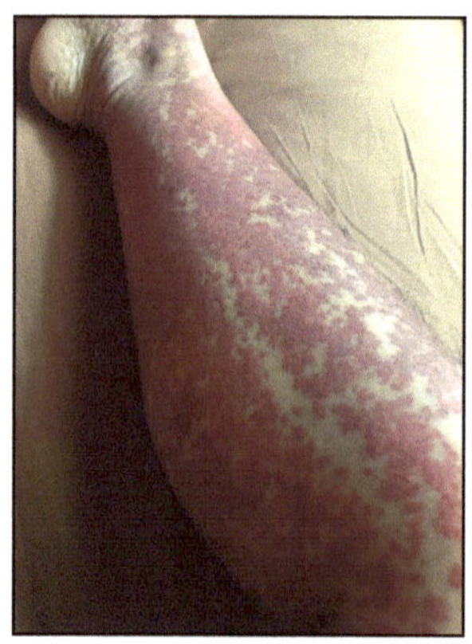

Tx:

Rheumatologic Labs

Anti-Cyclic Citrullinated Peptide: **RA**

RF: **RA**

Anti-dsDNA: **SLE**

Anti-GBM: **Goodpasture's**

Anti-Endomysial: **Celiac**

Anti-Histone: **Drug-induced SLE**

Anti-Smith: **SLE**

Anti-Jo: **Polymyositis, dermatomyositis**

Anti-Mi2: **Dermatomyositis**

Anti-Ro (SSA): **Sjögren's**

Anti-La (SSB): **Sjögren's**

Anti-SCL - 70: **Scleroderma (diffuse)**

Anti-Centromere: **CREST**

Anti-TPO: **Hashimotos**

Anti-TSI: **Grave's**

Anti-Mitochondrial: **Primary biliary cirrhosis**

pANCA: **Churg-Strauss, IBD, microscopic polyangiitis**

cANCA: **Wegener's**

HLA-B27:**(PAIR)psoriatic arthritis, ankylosing spondy, IBD, reactive arthritis**

Medications

________________: MOA = ____

Indication(s)=____

Side Effects = ____

Types/ Examples = ____

________________: MOA = ____

Indication(s)=____

Side Effects = ____

Types/ Examples = ____

________________: MOA = ____

Indication(s)=____

Side Effects = ____

Types/ Examples = ____

________________: MOA = ____

Indication(s)=____

Side Effects = ____

Types/ Examples = ____

________________: MOA = ____

Indication(s)=____

Side Effects = ____

Types/ Examples = ____

Medications

________________: **MOA =** ________________________________

Indication(s)=________________________________

Side Effects = ________________________________

Types/ Examples = ________________________________

________________: **MOA =** ________________________________

Indication(s)=________________________________

Side Effects = ________________________________

Types/ Examples = ________________________________

________________: **MOA =** ________________________________

Indication(s)=________________________________

Side Effects = ________________________________

Types/ Examples = ________________________________

________________: **MOA =** ________________________________

Indication(s)=________________________________

Side Effects = ________________________________

Types/ Examples = ________________________________

________________: **MOA =** ________________________________

Indication(s)=________________________________

Side Effects = ________________________________

Types/ Examples = ________________________________

EENT

Eye Disorders

All physical exams should include vision testing

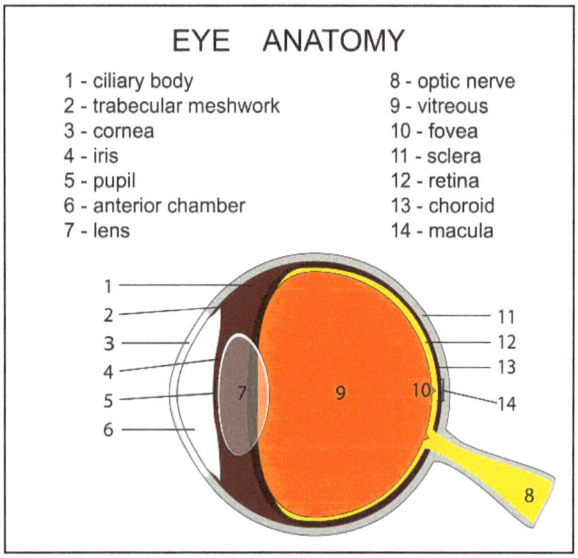

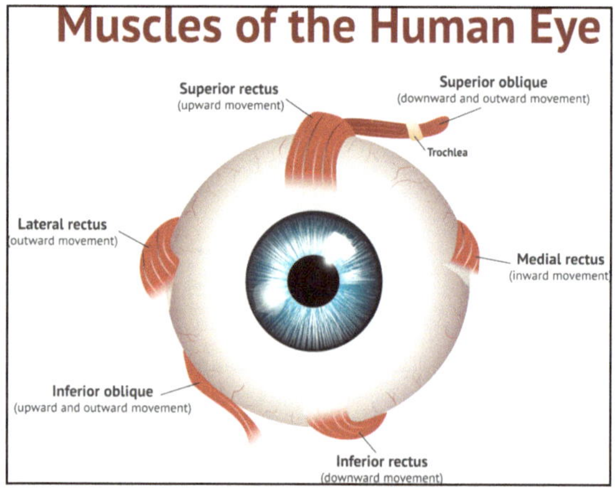

Blepharitis: **Inflammation of the eyelid margin**

Most common organism is S. aureus

Sx: Itching, burning, crusting of eye lids

PE:

Dx:

Tx:

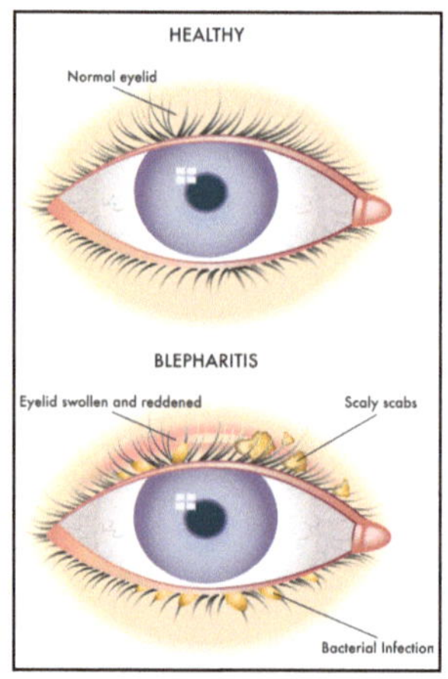

Blowout Fracture: **Trauma related**

Sx:

PE: Be sure to assess for possible inferior rectus entrapment!

Dx: CT with teardrop

Tx:

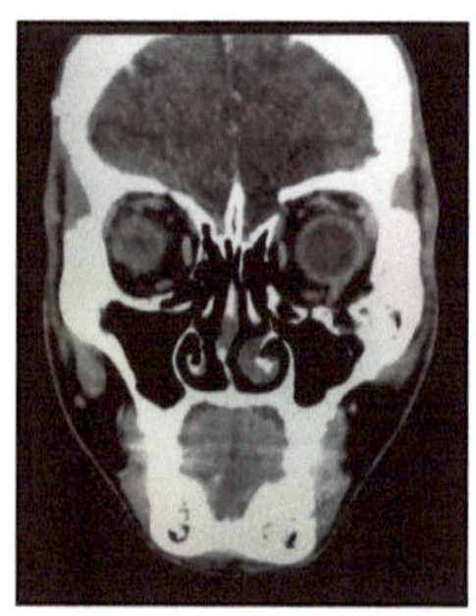

Cataract: Painless opacification of lens (usually due to aging)

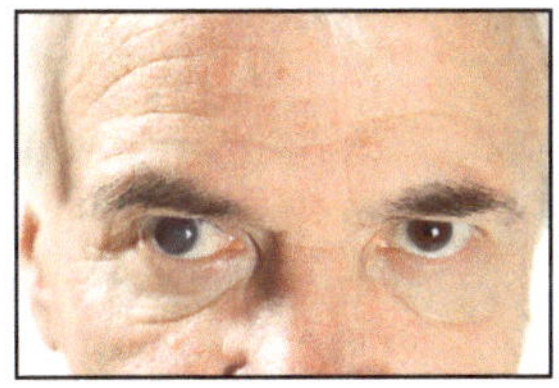

Sx: Blurred cloudy vision, decreased visual acuity

PE: Absent red reflex

Dx:

Tx:

Chalazion: Obstruction of meibomian sebaceous gland (can be chronic)

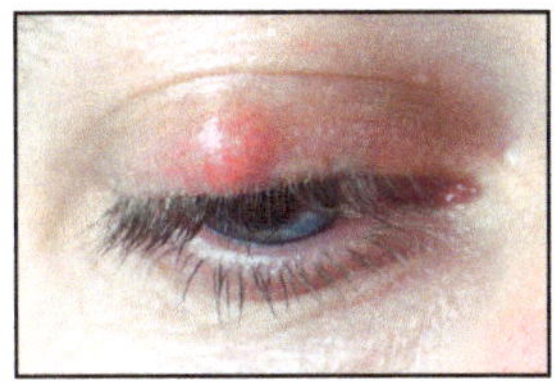

Sx: PAINLESS, lid swelling, slow growing

PE:

Dx:

Tx:

Hordeolum (Stye): Most common organism is S. aureus

Sx: PAINFUL, edema, pustule at eyelid margin, palpable tender nodule

PE:

Dx:

Tx:

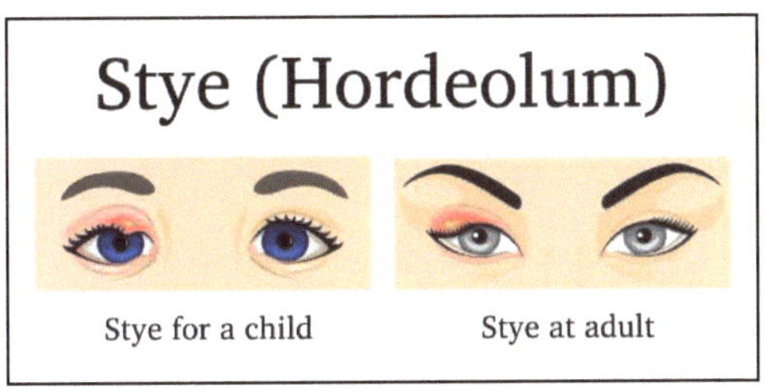

Chemical Burns: **Alkali is worse than acid –** ***EMERGENCY!!!***

Sx:

PE:

Dx: CBC, metabolic panel, carboxyhemoglobin, arterial blood gases

Tx:

Conjunctivitis:

Bacterial: **Most common organisms are S. aureus, S. pneumonia**

Sx: Crusting, purulent discharge

Dx:

Tx:

Viral: **Most common organism is Adenovirus**

Sx: Preauricular LAD, watery discharge

Dx:

Tx:

Allergic:

Sx: Stringy discharge, cobblestoned mucosa, bilateral erythema/irritation

Dx:

Tx:

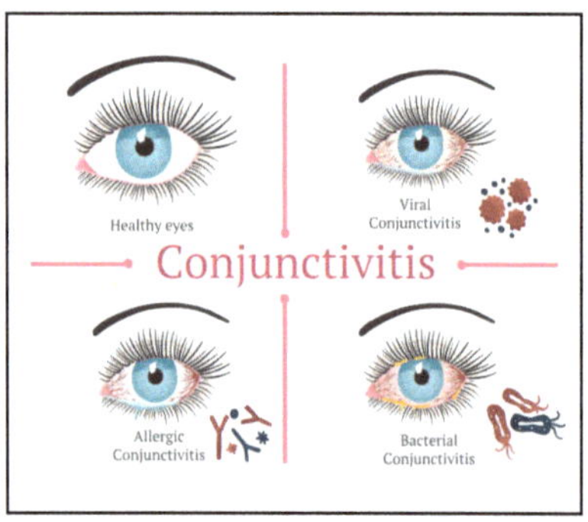

Corneal Abrasion:

Sx:

PE:

Dx: Fluorescein stain

Tx:

Corneal Ulcer (Keratitis):

Bacterial Keratitis:

Sx:

PE: Hazy cornea

Dx: Limbic flush

Tx:

HSV Keratitis:

Sx:

PE: Dendritic lesions

Dx: Conjunctival scrapings - microscope slide or culture

Tx:

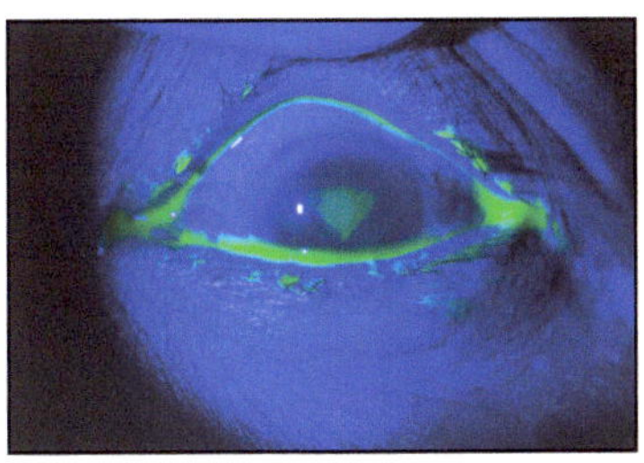

Corneal Abrasion

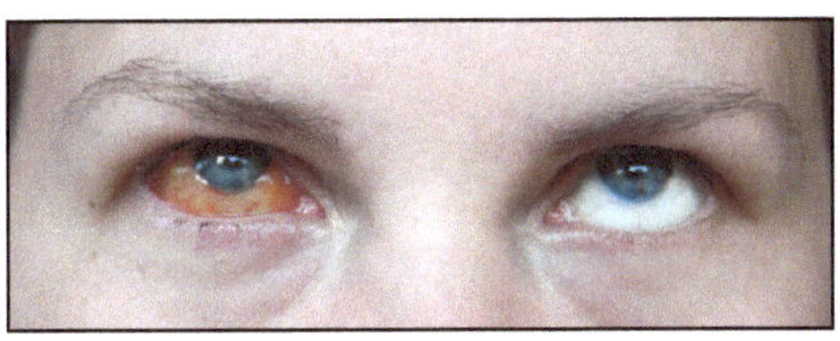

Bacterial Keratitis

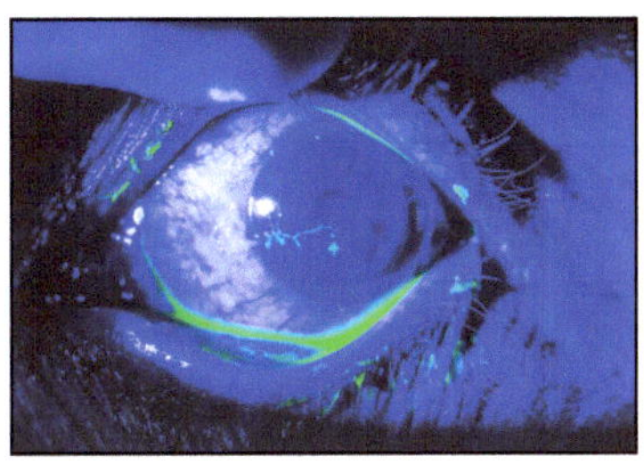

HSV Keratitis

Ectropion: Eyelid/lashes turn outward

Most common in elderly patients

Sx: Irritation, ocular dryness, eyelid sagging

PE:

Dx:

Tx:

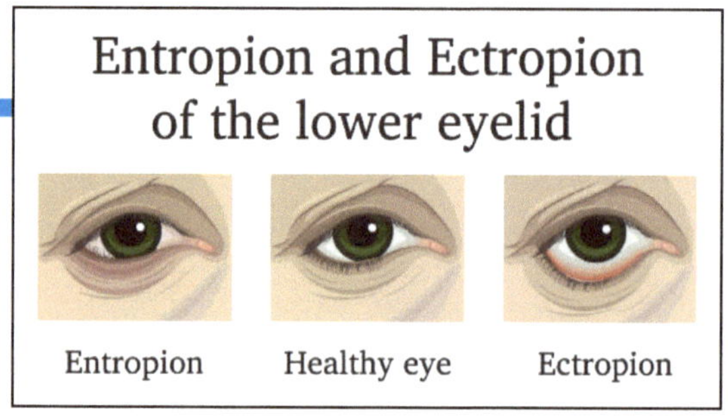

Entropion: Eyelid/lashes turn inward

Most common in elderly patients

Sx: Erythema, tearing, increased sensitivity

PE:

Dx:

Tx:

Globe Rupture: Outer eye membranes disrupted by Trauma - EMERGENCY!!!

Sx: Enophthalmos, conjunctival hemorrhage, teardrop or irregularly shaped pupil

PE:

Dx:

Tx:

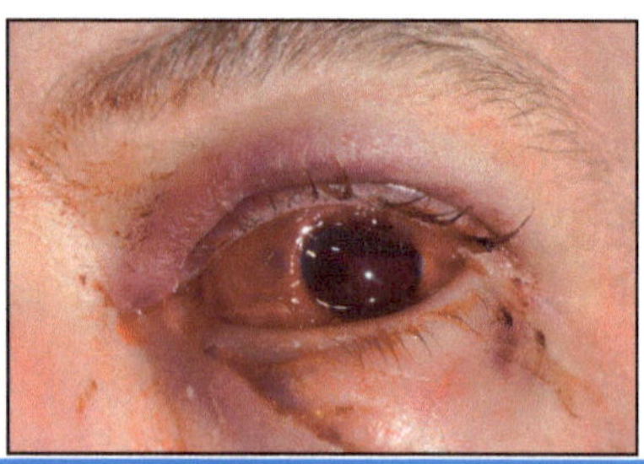

Glaucoma: Increased intraocular pressure, cupping, peripheral vision loss

Acute (Angle Closure Glaucoma):

Sx: Sudden onset, painful, erythematous eye with "steamy" cornea. Fixed mid-dilated pupil, halos in vision

PE:

Dx:

________________________________ Tx:

____

Chronic (Open Angle Glaucoma):

Sx: Slow onset without pain

PE:

Dx:

________________________________ Tx:

____

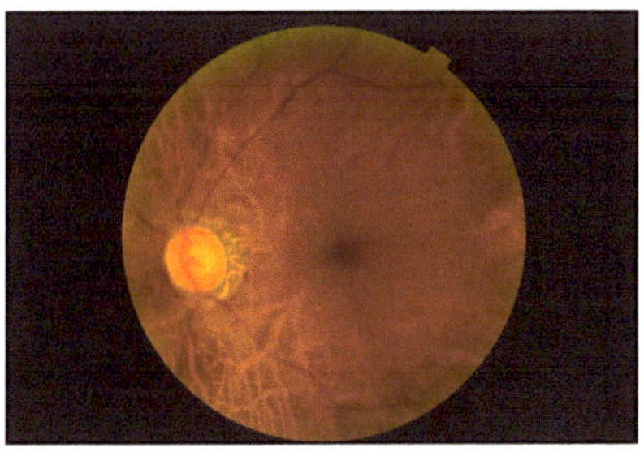

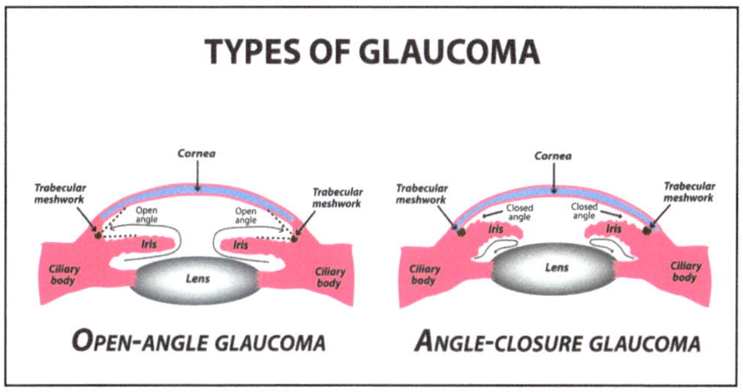

Hyphema:

Sx: Blood in anterior chamber, usually due to trauma

PE:

Dx:

____

____

____

Tx:

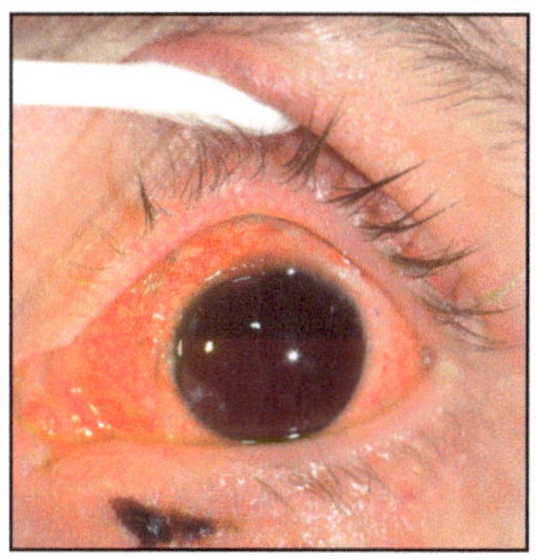

Macular Degeneration: **Most common cause of irreversible vision loss in the U.S.**

Sx: Central vision loss

PE: Dry - Drussen spots

Wet - Neovascularization with bleeding

Dx: Amsler grid:

Tx:

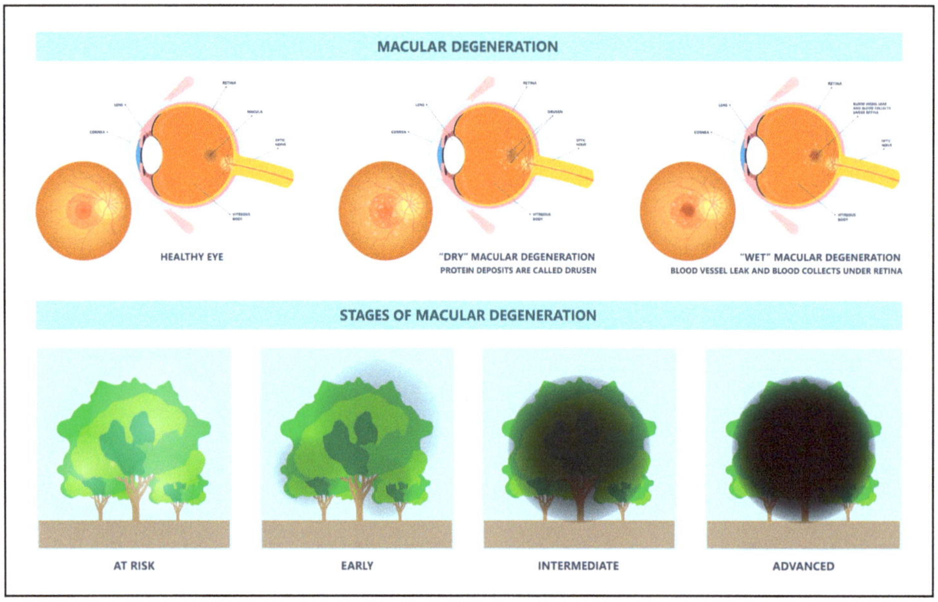

Optic Neuritis: **Associated with multiple sclerosis**

Sx: Vision loss, pain with movement, periorbital/retro-ocular pain

PE: Altered perception of color

Dx:

Tx:

Orbital (Septal) Cellulitis:

Sx:

PE:

Dx: CT with contrast of sinus and orbits

Tx:

Periorbital (Preseptal) Cellulitis: Eyelid infection

Sx: No pain with eye movement, eyelid erythema & edema

PE:

Dx:

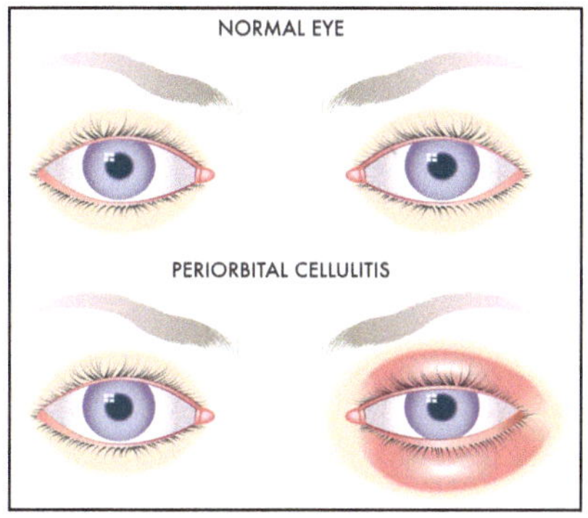

Tx:

Papilledema: Optic nerve swelling

Most common cause is idiopathic

Sx:

PE:

Dx: Visual field testing, fundoscopy, MRI + LP to rule out mass

Tx:

Pterygium:

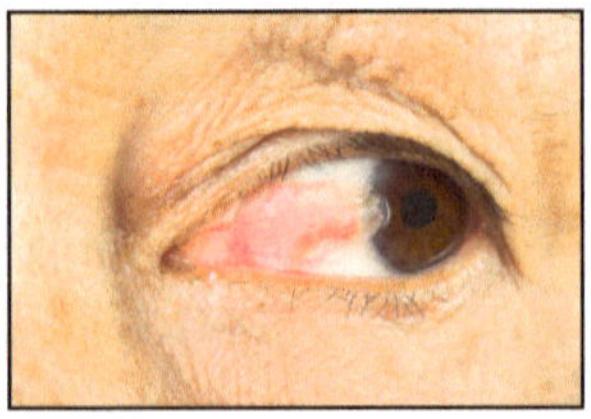

Sx: Wing shaped conjunctival growth over cornea/pupil

PE:

Dx:

Tx:

Retinal Detachment:

Sx: "Curtain drop", floaters, painless & sudden vision loss. EMERGENCY!!!

PE:

Dx: Fundoscopy

Tx:

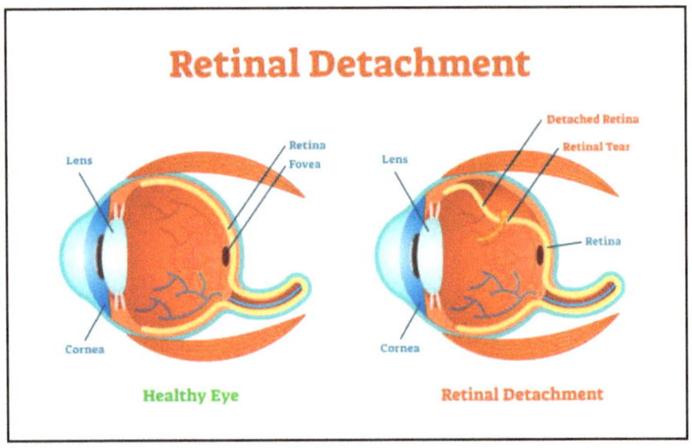

Central Retinal Artery Occlusion:

Sx: Amaurosis fugax

PE: Cherry red macula

Dx:

Tx:

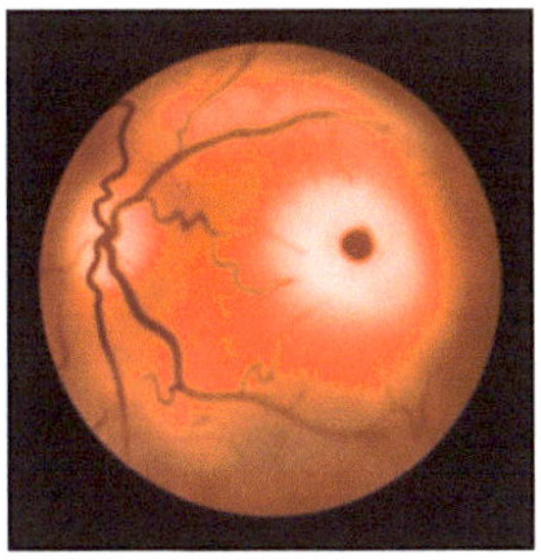

Central Retinal Vein Occlusion:

Sx: Sudden vision loss

PE:

Dx:

Tx:

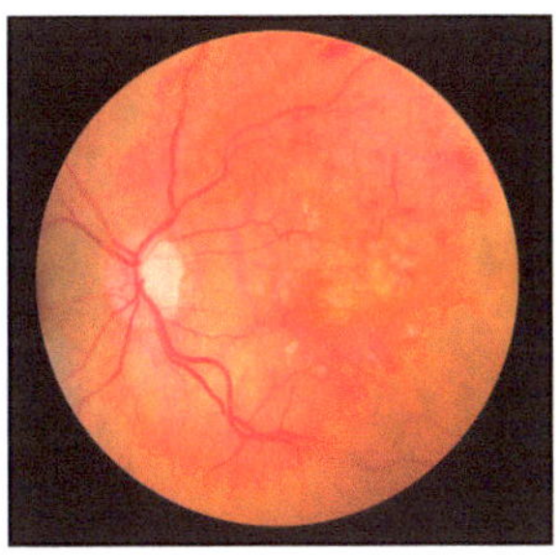

Retinopathy:

Diabetic (Non-Proliferative):

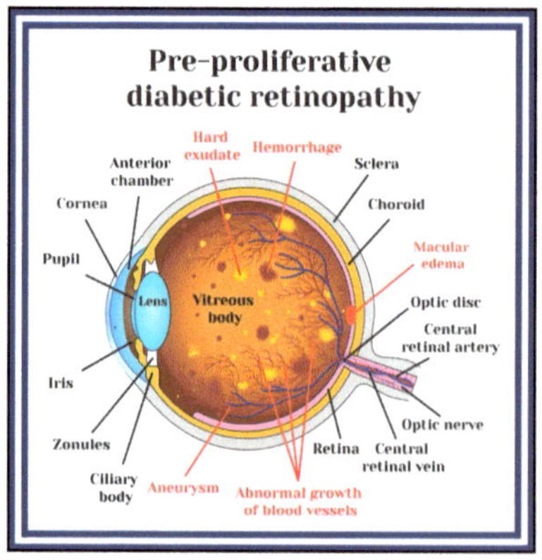

Sx: New, permanent vision loss

PE: Flame hemorrhages

Dx:

Tx:

Diabetic (Proliferative): Neovascularization

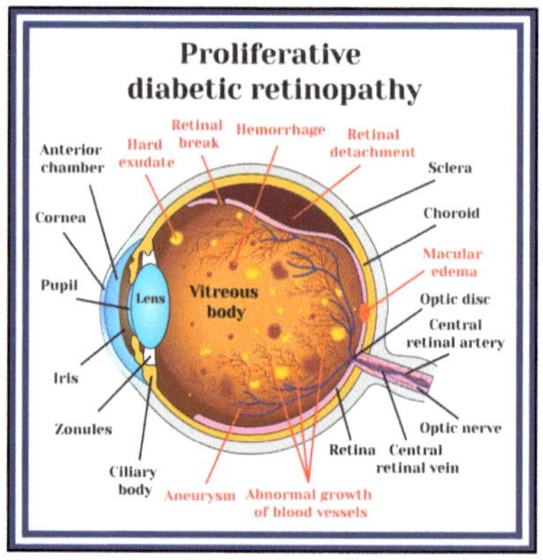

Sx:

PE: AV nicking, cotton wool spots, concern for papilledema

Dx: Field stereoscopic fundus photography

Tx:

Hypertensive:

Sx: Vision loss

PE: Narrow arteries (copper/silver wire)

Dx:

Tx:

Strabismus:

Sx:

PE:

Dx: Cover/uncover test

Tx:

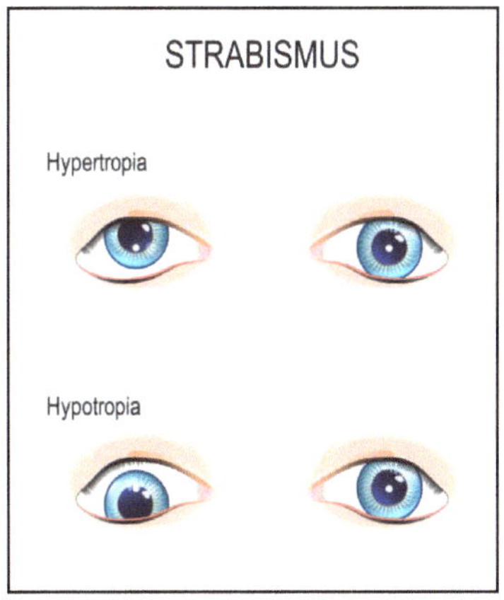

Uveitis: Inflammation of uvea

Anterior (Iritis): Most common cause is infectious

Sx: Pain, erythema, vision loss

PE:

Dx:

Tx:

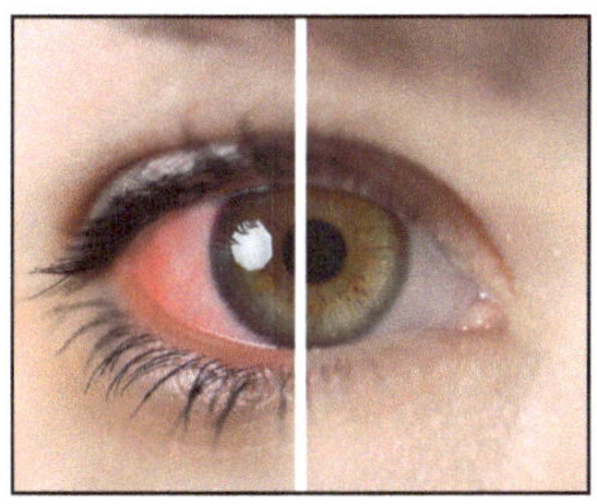

Posterior (Chorioretinitis): Most common cause is systemic inflammation

Sx:

PE:

Dx: Clinical

Tx:

Hyperopia: "Farsighted"

Sx:

PE:

Dx:

Tx:

Myopia: "Nearsighted"

Sx:

PE:

Dx:

Tx:

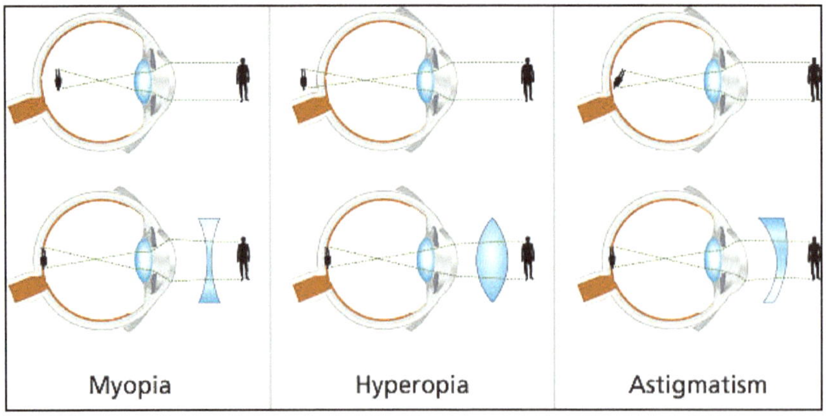

Visual Pathways Defects

Ear Disorders

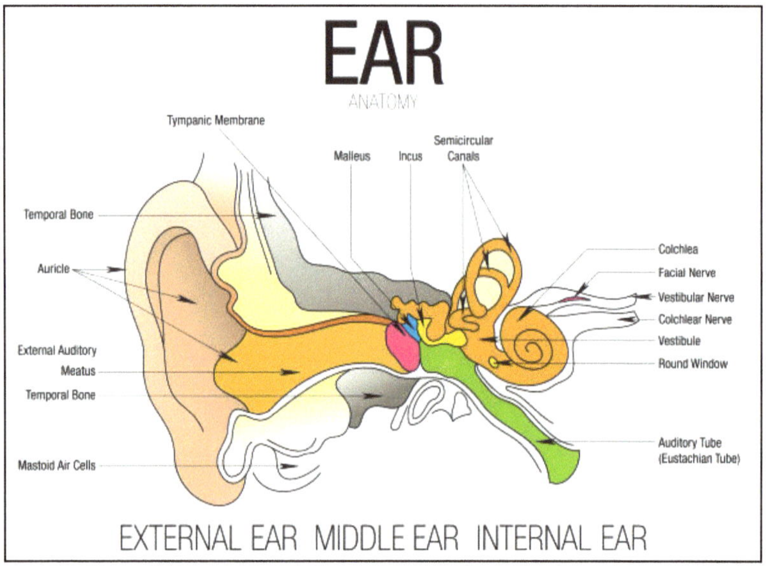

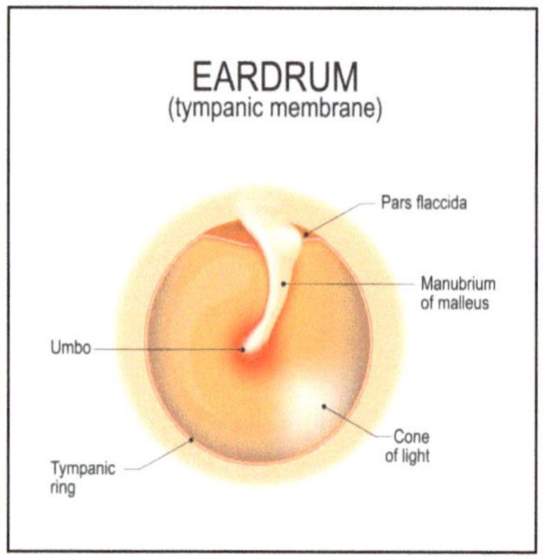

Acute Otitis Media:

Common organisms: S. pneumoniae, H. influenzae, Group A Strep

Sx:

PE: Effusion, bulging TM, decreased movement, purulent fluid behind TM, no light reflex, dull

Dx:

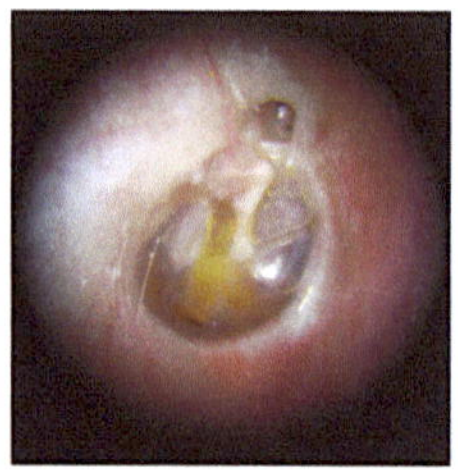

Tx:

Chronic Otitis Media: Tympanic membrane with perforation or otorrhea

Sx: Otorrhea, pain, sudden "pop"

PE: Possible opening in TM

Dx:

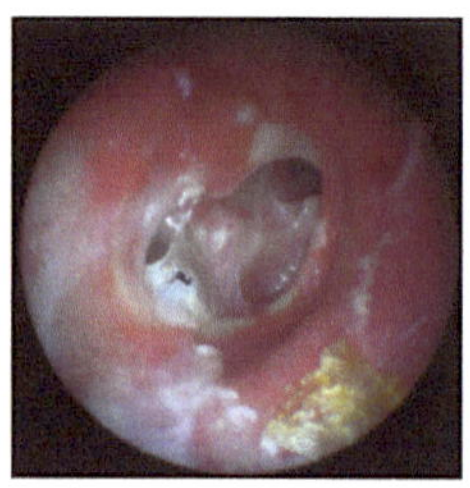

Tx:

Mastoiditis: Infection in mastoid air cells of the temporal bone

Most common cause: Chronic otitis media (Pseudomonas)

Sx:

PE:

Dx: CT with contrast

Tx:

Acute Otitis Externa: "Swimmer's ear". Most common organism is Pseudomonas

Sx: Ear pain, decreased hearing

PE:

Dx: Otoscope

Tx:

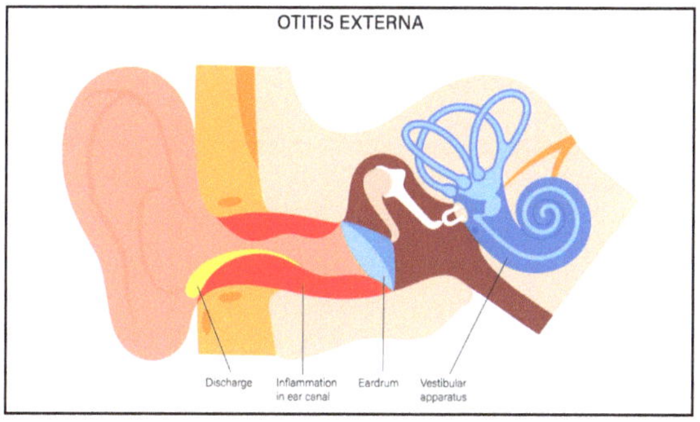

Malignant Otitis Externa: Osteomyelitis at the skull base

Most common cause: Patients who are immunocomproised or have diabetes mellitus

Sx:

PE:

Dx: Otoscope visualization shows edema & erythema of ear canal
CT/MRI/Biopsy

Tx:

Acoustic Neuroma: Vestibular schwannoma CN VIII

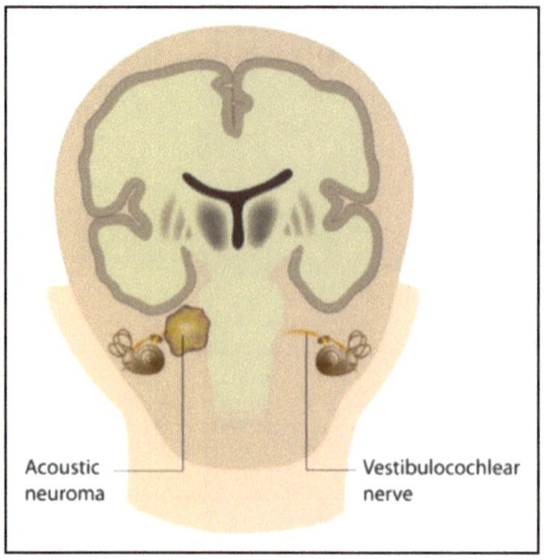

Sx:

PE:

Dx: Audiogram, gadolinium-enhanced MRI with contrast

Tx:

Cerumen Impaction:

Sx: Diminished hearing, fullness of ear, possible otorrhea

PE:

Dx: Otoscope

Tx:

Cholesteatoma: Keratinized desquamated epithelium

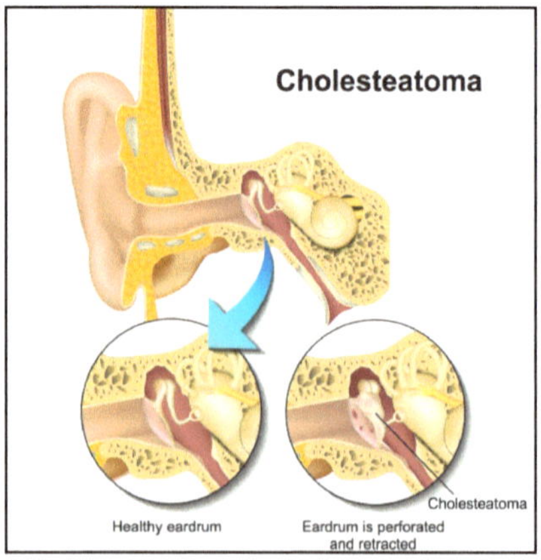

Sx:

PE:

Dx: Otoscope visualization shows granulation tissue

Tx:

Eustachian Tube Dysfunction: Often found with viral URI, allergic rhinitis, or barotrauma

Sx: Hearing loss, aural fullness, complaints of "can't pop ears"

PE:

Dx:

Tx:

Hearing Loss

Conductive Hearing Loss: Most common cause is cerumen impaction

Sx:

PE:

Dx: Weber lateralizes to affected side. Rinne shows bone conduction > air conduction

Tx:

Sensorineural Hearing Loss: Most common cause of hearing loss in adults

Sx:

PE:

Dx: Weber lateralizes to "good" ear. Rinne shows air conduction > bone conduction

Tx:

Auricular Hematoma: Usually related to trauma

Sx: Physical deformity, swelling and/or bruising of the auricle

PE:

Dx:

Tx:

Otosclerosis: **Abnormal bony overgrowth of stapes**

Sx: Slow, progressive conductive hearing loss and tinnitus

PE:

Dx:

______________________________ Tx:

____

____

Tinnitus: **Ringing in ears**

Sx:

PE:

Dx: Audiometry

______________________________ Tx:

____

____

Tympanic Membrane Perforation:

Sx: Otorrhea, ear pain, decreased hearing in affected ear

PE:

Dx:

______________________________ Tx:

____

____

Tympanosclerosis: **Scarring of the eradrum**

Sx: Small white area on TM (usually from perforation or tubes)

PE:

Dx:

______________________________ Tx:

____

____

Vertigo

Peripheral: Vestibular

Sx: False sense of motion (or exaggerated sense of motion)

PE:

Dx:

Tx:

____

____

____

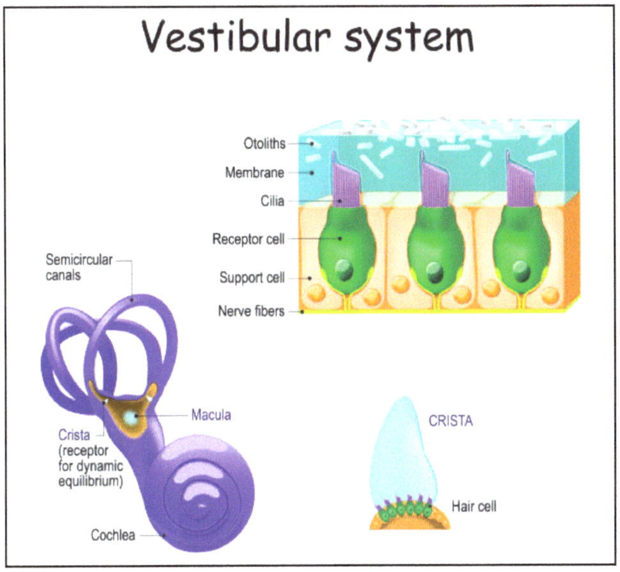

Central: Brainstem & cerebellum

More common in patients with multiple sclerosis & ischemic posterior circulation stroke

Sx:

PE:

Dx: Gait issues, positive CNS signs, non-fatigable vertical nystagmus

Tx:

____

____

____

Benign Paroxysmal Positional Vertigo (BPPV): **Displaced otoliths (small calcium carbonate crystals on cilia)**

Sx: Lasting second to minutes

PE:

Dx: + Dix-Hallpike (fatigable nystagmus)

____ **Tx:**

____

____

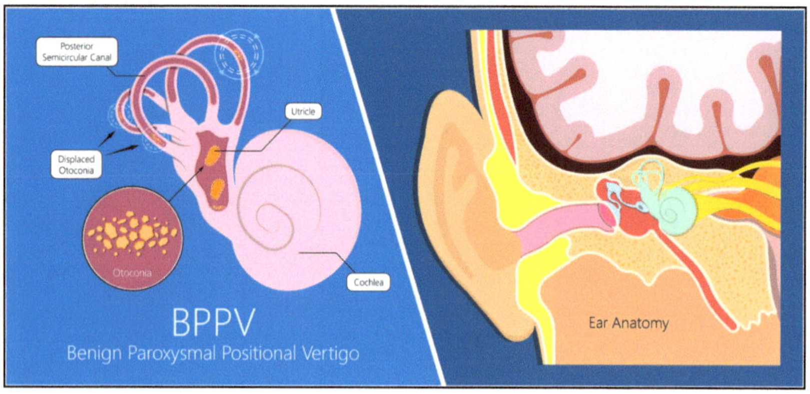

Ménière's Disease: **Excess endolymph in inner ear**

Sx: Vertigo for minutes to hours, low frequency sensorineural hearing loss + tinnitus + pressure

PE:

Dx: Transtympanic electrocochleography, caloric testing

____ **Tx:**

____

____

Vestibular Neuritis: **Inflammation of vestibular portion of CN VIII**

Common causes: Viral infection

Sx: Lasting days to weeks

PE:

Dx: Clinical, MRI to rule out other possible causes

Tx:

Labyrinthitis: **Inflammation of vestibular & cochlear portion of CN VIII**

Sx: Symptoms of vestibular neuritis + unilateral hearing loss + tinnitus

PE:

Dx:

Tx:

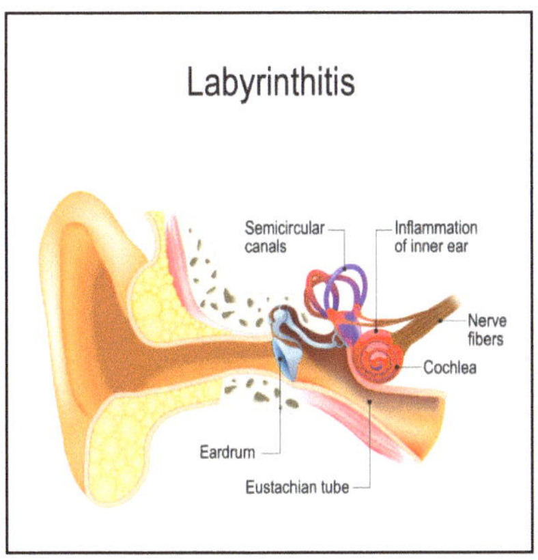

Nose/Sinus Disorders

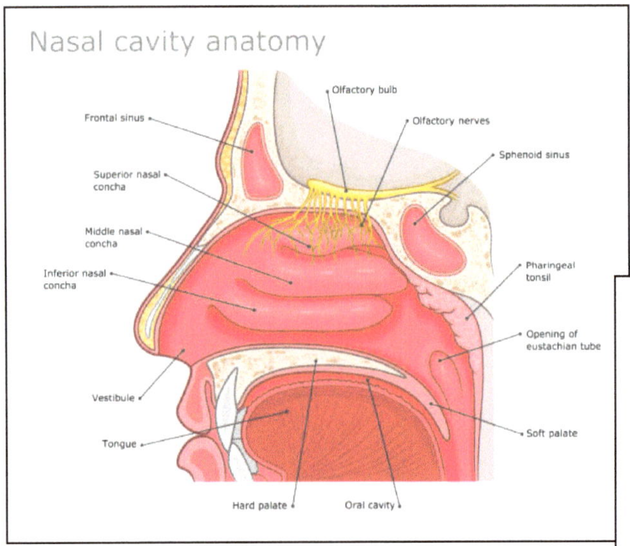

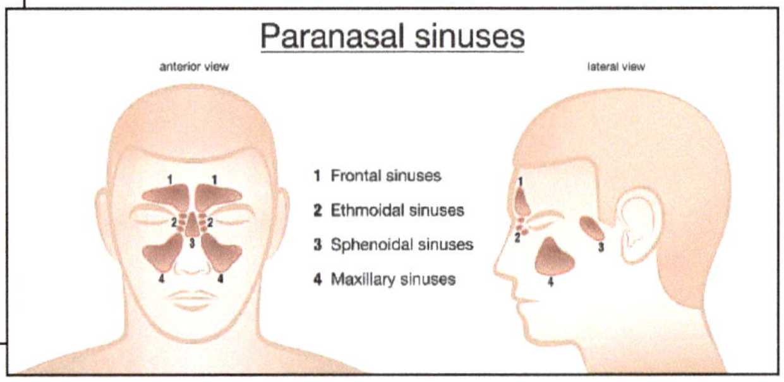

Rhinosinusitis (Acute Sinusitis): **More common in maxillary sinuses**

Common organisms: S. pneumoniae, H. influenzae, Group A strep

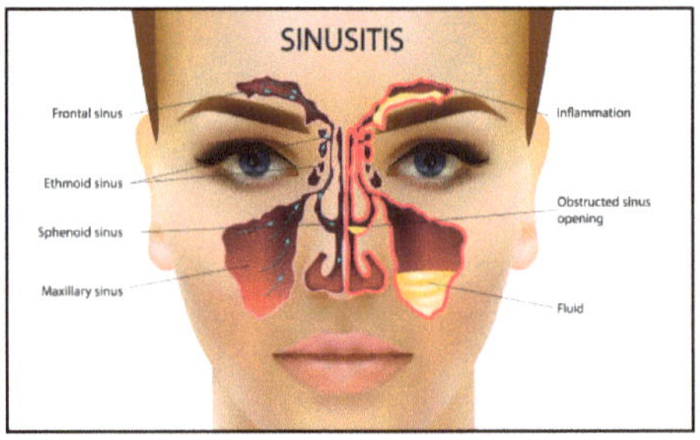

Sx: Rhinorrhea, sinus pain, referred dental pain

PE:

Dx:

Tx:

Chronic Sinusitis: **12+ weeks of symptoms**

Sx: Same as acute sinusitis

PE:

Dx: CT

Tx:

Allergic Rhinitis: IgE

Sx:

PE: Pale, blue, boggy, nares with cobblestoning. May have nasal polyps

Dx: Trial of antihistamine or intranasal corticosteroid, allergy testing

Tx:

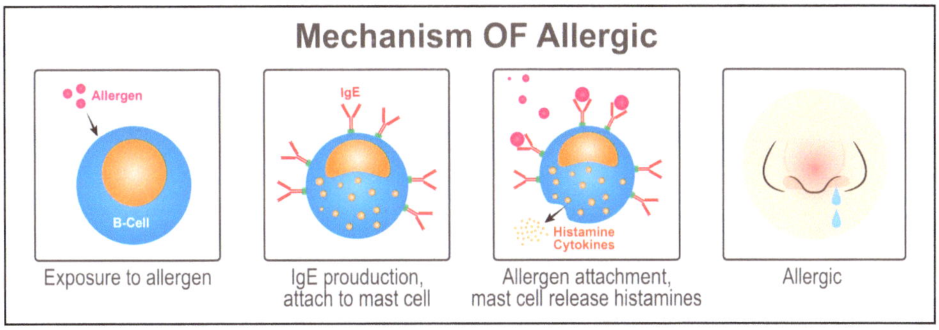

Foreign Body: Most common in kids

Sx: Foul smelling nares, epistaxis, mucopurulent discharge

PE:

Dx:

Tx:

Nasal Polyps: More common in patients with allergic rhinitis

Samter's Triad: Asthma, nasal polyps, Aspirin/NSAID sensitivity/allergy

Sx:

PE:

Dx:

Tx:

Epistaxis

Anterior: Kiesselbach's plexus (more common with trauma)

Sx:

PE:

Dx: Clinical

Tx:

____

____

____

Posterior: Sphenopalatine artery (posterior pharynx)

Sx: Blood in both nares and posterior pharynx

PE:

Dx:

Tx:

____

____

____

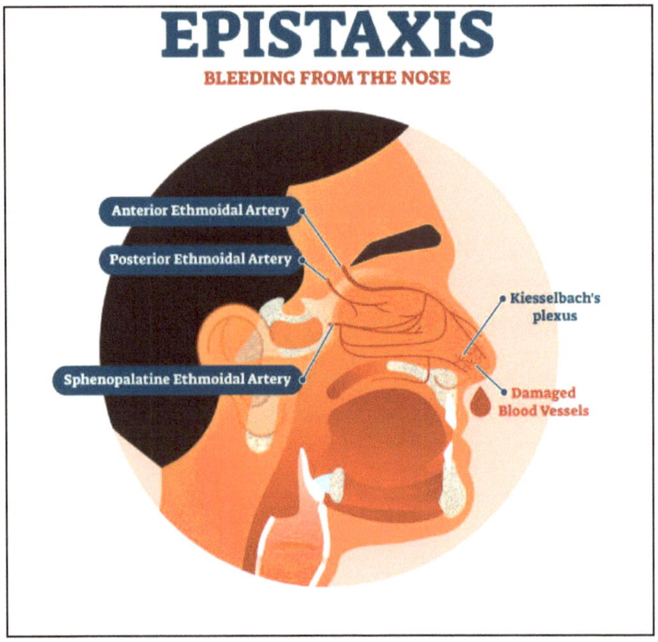

Throat Disorders

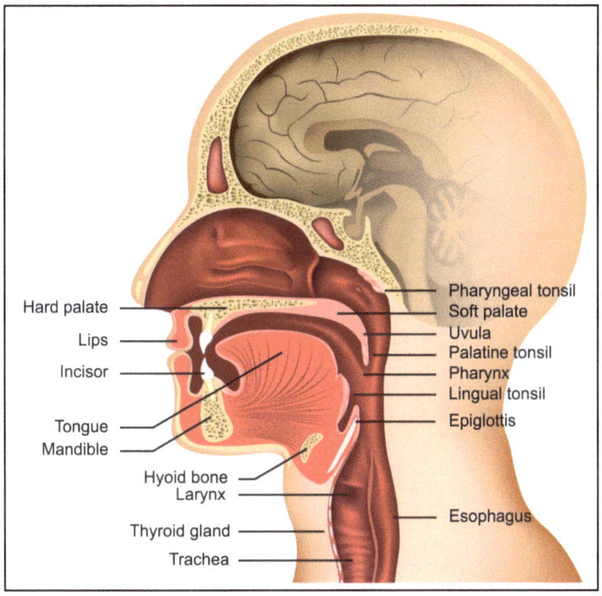

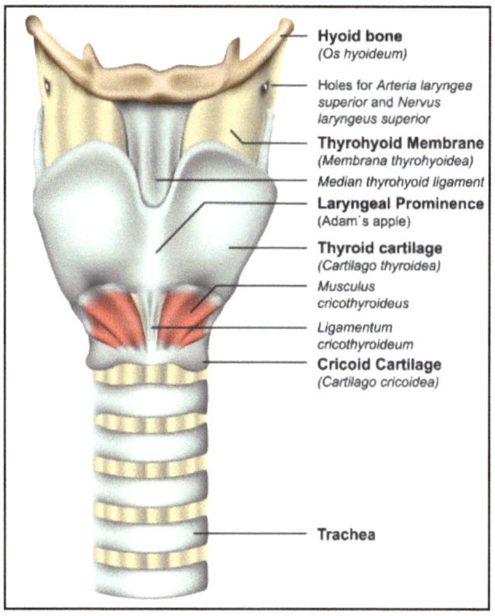

Acute Pharyngitis/Tonsillitis: Bacterial (Group A Strep)

Most common overall cause is viral

Complications:

Scarlet fever:

Rheumatic fever:

Sx: Scarlatina rash, exudates, no cough, sore throat, difficulty swallowing

PE:

Dx:

____

____

____

Tx:

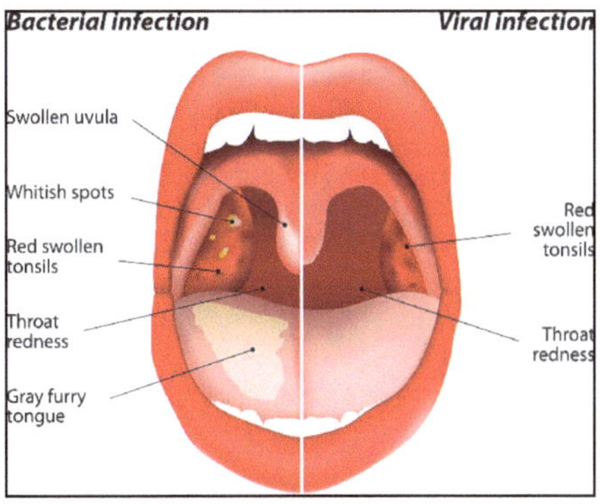

Aphthous Ulcer: **"Canker sore"**

Sx: Painful, shallow ulcer with yellow, white or grey central exudate and surrounding erythema

PE:

Dx:

______________________________ **Tx:**

____

____

Croup (Parainfluenza):

Sx: Barking cough, inspiratory stridor, hoarseness

PE:

Dx:

______________________________ **Tx:**

____

____

Epiglottitis: **Most common cause is H. flu**

Sx: Dysphagia, inspiratory stridor, tripod, drooling, muffled "hot potato" voice

PE:

Dx:

______________________________ **Tx:**

____

____

Laryngitis:

Common causes: Viral upper respiratory infection, bacterial infection, trauma

Sx: Hoarseness, aphonia, dry scratchy throat, runny nose, cough, sore throat

PE:

Dx:

______________________________ Tx:

____

____

Ludwig's Angina: Cellulitis of sublingual or submaxillary space

Most common cause: Dental infection

Sx: Swelling, "woody" induration, pus

PE:

Dx:

______________________________ Tx:

____

____

Oral Candidiasis (Thrush):

Sx:

PE:

Dx: Clinical. KOH shows budding yeast & pseudo hyphae

______________________________ Tx:

____

____

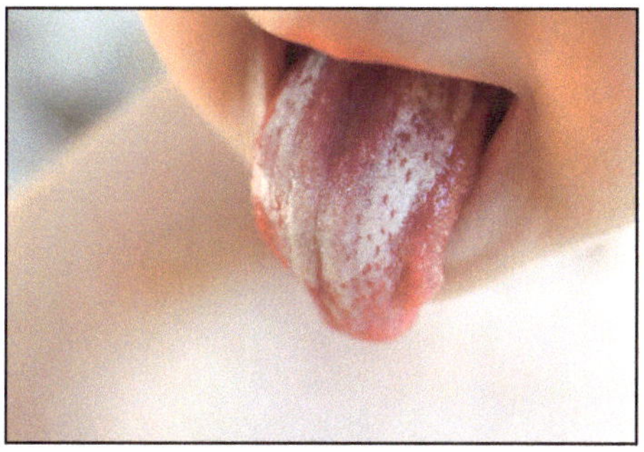

Erythroplakia: **High risk of malignant transformation**

Risk Factor: Cigarette smoking

Sx: Painless, erythematous, soft, velvety, patch in mouth

PE:

Dx:

____ **Tx:**

____

____

Oral Leukoplakia: **Caused by Epstein-Barr virus. More common in immunocompromised patients**

Sx: Painless white plaque along lateral tongue border or buccal mucosa

PE:

Dx:

____ **Tx:**

____

____

Oral Hairy Leukoplakia:

Sx: Painless, erythematous, soft, velvety, patch in mouth

PE:

Dx:

____ **Tx:**

____

____

Oral Lichen Planus: **Autoimmune or Hepatits C (most common causes)**

Sx: Lacy reticular leukoplakia (Wickham striae), erythematous ulcers

PE:

Dx:

Tx:

Peritonsillar Abscess:

Most common organisms: Group A Strep, S. aureus, polymicrobial

Sx: "Hot potato" voice, drooling, trismus, uvula to contralateral side

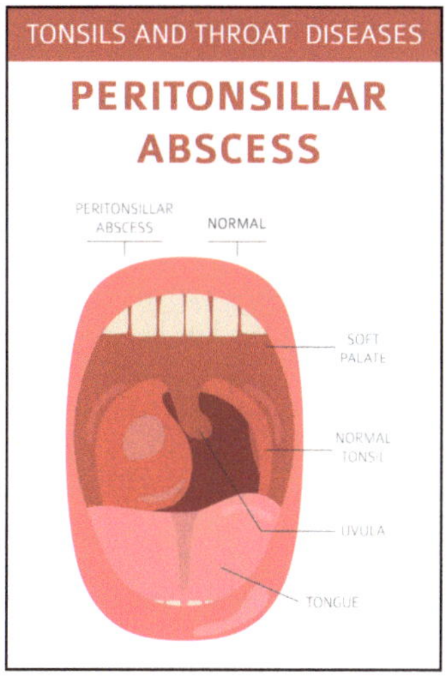

PE:

Dx:

Tx:

Retropharyngeal Abscess:

Sx: Difficulty and pain with swallowing, fever, stiff neck, drooling, difficulty breathing

PE:

Dx:

Tx:

Parotitis/Sialadenitis: **Inflammation of salivary glands**

Most common infectious cause:

Most common bacterial cause:

Sx: Sudden onset, dysphagia, trismus. Tenderness, swelling, and purulent discharge of salivary glands

PE:

Dx:

Tx:

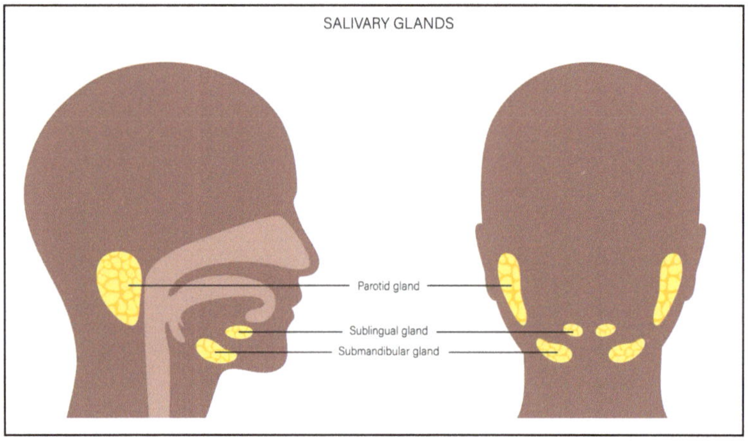

Sialolithiasis: **Most common at Wharton's ducts (submandibular gland) and Stensen's duct (parotid gland)**

Sx: Post prandial salivary gland pain and swelling

PE:

Dx:

Tx:

EENT Neoplasms

Nasopharyngeal Carcinomas: **Associated with tobacco, EtOH, EBV**

Sx: Difficulty speaking, breathing, hearing

PE:

Dx:

Tx:

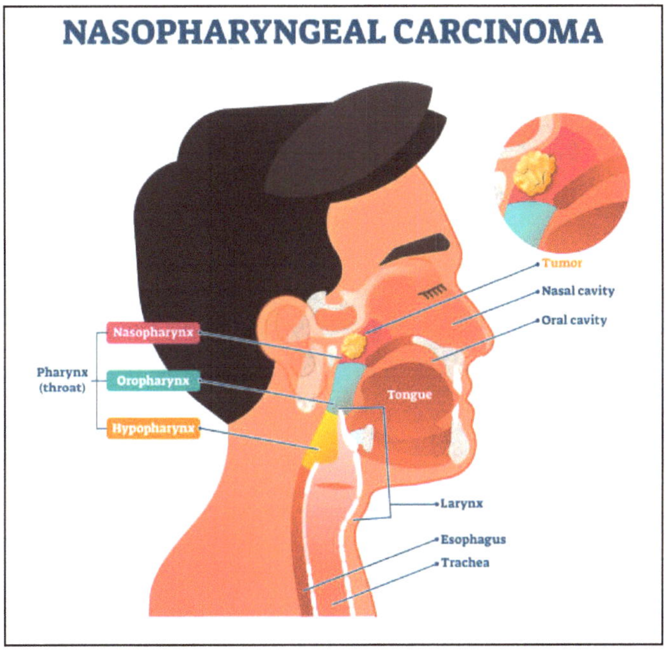

Herpes Simplex Virus 1: ***In ID***

Medications

____________________: MOA = ____________________
Indication(s)= ____________________
Side Effects = ____________________
Types/ Examples = ____________________

____________________: MOA = ____________________
Indication(s)= ____________________
Side Effects = ____________________
Types/ Examples = ____________________

____________________: MOA = ____________________
Indication(s)= ____________________
Side Effects = ____________________
Types/ Examples = ____________________

____________________: MOA = ____________________
Indication(s)= ____________________
Side Effects = ____________________
Types/ Examples = ____________________

____________________: MOA = ____________________
Indication(s)= ____________________
Side Effects = ____________________
Types/ Examples = ____________________

Medications

________________: MOA = ________________________________

Indication(s)=________________________________

Side Effects = ________________________________

Types/ Examples = ________________________________

____

____

________________: MOA = ________________________________

Indication(s)=________________________________

Side Effects = ________________________________

Types/ Examples = ________________________________

____

____

________________: MOA = ________________________________

Indication(s)=________________________________

Side Effects = ________________________________

Types/ Examples = ________________________________

____

____

________________: MOA = ________________________________

Indication(s)=________________________________

Side Effects = ________________________________

Types/ Examples = ________________________________

____

____

________________: MOA = ________________________________

Indication(s)=________________________________

Side Effects = ________________________________

Types/ Examples = ________________________________

____

____

Appendix

Cardiology 1

Inflammatory Cardiac Disorders 2
- Pericarditis 2
- Dressler's Syndrome 2
- Pericardial Effusion 2
- Cardiac Tamponade 3
- Myocarditis 3
- Endocarditis 4

Valvular Disorders 5
- Aortic Stenosis 5
- Aortic Regurgitation 5
- Mitral Stenosis 6
- Mitral Regurgitation 6
- Mitral Valve Prolapse 6
- Pulmonary Stenosis 7
- Pulmonary Regurgitation 7
- Tricuspid Stenosis 8
- Tricuspid Regurgitation 8
- Rheumatic Fever 8

Systolic Murmurs 9

Diastolic Murmurs 9
- Innocent Murmurs 10
- Still's Murmur 10
- Cervical Venous Hum 10
- **EKG (Labeled) 11**
- Murmur Vocabulary 11

Acute Coronary Syndrome 12
- Stable Angina 12
- Unstable Angina 12
- Prinzmetal Angina 12
- NSTEMI 13
- STEMI 13

Acute Myocardial Infarction 14
- Anterior MI 14
- Inferior & Right Ventricle MI 14
- Lateral MI 14
- Posterior MI 14
  - *Beck's triad 14

Post MI Care 15

Dysrhythmias & Conduction Disorders 16
- 1st Degree Heart Block 16
- 2nd Degree Heart Block (Mobitz I) 16
- 2nd Degree Heart Block (Mobitz II) 16
- 3rd Degree Heart Block 16
- Bundle Branch Block 17
- Right Bundle Branch Block (RBBB) 17
- Left Bundle Branch Block (LBBB) 17
- Sick Sinus Syndrome 18
- **Premature Beats 18**
  - Premature Atrial Contraction (PAC) 18
  - Premature Ventricular Contraction (PVC) 18
  - Premature Junctional Contraction (PJC) 18
- **Sinus Arrythmia 19**
- Atrial Fibrillation 19
- Atrial Flutter 19
- Supraventricular Tachycardia (SVT) 20
- Wolff - Parkinson - White (WPW) Syndrome 20
- Long QT Syndrome 20
- Ventricular Tachycardia (VT) 21
- Torsades de Pointes 21
- Ventricular Fibrillation 21

Vascular Disorders 22
- Chronic Peripheral Arterial Disease 22
- Acute Peripheral Arterial Disease 22
- Abdominal Aortic Aneurysm 23
- Thoracic Aortic Aneurysm 23
- Aortic Dissection 24
- Arteriovenous Malformation 24
- Giant Cell (Temporal) Arteritis 25
- Deep Vein Thrombosis (DVT) 25
- Superficial Vein Thrombophlebitis (Phlebitis) 25
- Acute Mesenteric Ischemia 26
- Chronic Mesenteric Ischemia 26
- Buerger's Disease (Thromboangiitis Obliterans) 27
- Raynaud's 27
- Varicose Veins 27
- Venous Insufficiency 28
- Carotid Occlusive Disease 28

Hypertension, Cardiomyopathy, & Heart Failure 29
- Essential Hypertension 29
- Secondary Hypertension 29
- Hypertensive Urgency 30

Hypertensive Emergency 30
Malignant Hypertension 30
Hypotension 31
Cardiogenic Shock 31
Orthostatic Hypotension 31
Vasovagal Hypotension 31
Cardiomyopathy 32
Dilated Cardiomyopathy 33
Hypertrophic Cardiomyopathy 33
Restrictive Cardiomyopathy 343
Heart Failure 34
Left Ventricular Systolic Heart Failure 34
Left Ventricular Diastolic Heart Failure 34
Right Heart Failure 34
Congenital Heart Defects 35
Atrial Septal Defect (ASD) 35
Ventricular Septal Defect (VSD) 35
Coarctation of Aorta 36
Patent Ductus Arteriosus 36
Tetralogy of Fallot 37
Atrial Myxoma 37
Lipid Disorders 38
Hypercholesterolemia 38
Hypertriglyceridemia 38
Hypertension Medications 39
Alpha/Beta blockers 39
ACE Inhibitors 40
ARBs 40
Renin Inhibitors 40
CCBs 41
Direct Acting Vasodilators 42
Nitrates 42
Diuretics 43
Anticoagulation 44
Direct Oral Anticoagulants 44
Antiplatelets 44
Clotting Cascade 45
Platelet Activation 45
Hypercholesteremia Medications 46
Statins 46
PCSK9 46
Bile Acid Sequestrants 46
Niacin 46
Ezetimibe 46
Fibrates 46

Pulmonology 54
Chronic Obstructive Pulmonary Disease 57
Chronic Bronchitis 57
Emphysema 57
Asthma 58
Asthma (Obstructive) Medications 61
Restrictive Pulmonary Disease 62
Idiopathic Pulmonary Fibrosis 62
Pneumoconiosis 63
Asbestosis 63
Silicosis 63
Berylliosis 63
Coal Worker's Pneumoconiosis (Black Lung) 64
Sarcoidosis 64
Infectious Pulmonary Disorders 65
Acute Bronchiolitis (RSV) 65
Acute Bronchitis 65
Pertussis "Whooping Cough" 66
Influenza A & B 66
Pneumonia 67
Bacterial 68
Pneumococcal Pneumonia 68
M. Catarrhalis 68
Haemophilius Influenzae 68
Atypical 68
Chlamydia Pneumoniae 68
Legionella 68
Mycoplasma Pneumoniae 68
Hospital Acquired 69
Pseudomonas 69
Other Pneumonia 69
Aspiration Pneumonia 69
Viral Pneumonia 69
Tuberculosis 70
Bronchiectasis 71
Lung Abscess 71
Empyema 71
Pulmonic Nodules & Neoplasms 72
Small Cell Lung Cancer 72
Squamous Cell Lung Cancer 72
Large Cell Lung Cancer 72
Adenocarcinoma 73
Pulmonary Nodules 73
Pleural Diseases 74
Pleural Effusions 74

Pneumothorax 75
Pulmonary Circulation Disorders 76
Pulmonary Embolism (PE) 76
Pulmonary Hypertension 77
Sleep Apnea 78
Other Pulmonary Disorders 79
Acute Respiratory Distress Syndrome (ARDS) 79
Samter's Triad 80
Cystic Fibrosis (CF) 80
Foreign Body Aspiration 81
Atelectasis 81
Obesity Hypoventilation Syndrome 82

Acute Epiglottitis: In EENT
Croup (Parainfluenza): In EENT
Polyangiitis (Wegener's, Churg - Strauss): In Renal
Fungal Pneumonia: In ID
Mycobacterium Avium Complex: In ID
Carcinoid Tumors: In GI

Gastrointestinal 89

Esophageal 90
Eosinophilic Esophagitis (EoE) 90
Pill Induced Esophagitis 90
Infectious Esophagitis 90
Non - Infectious Esophagitis 91
Gastroesophageal Reflux Disease (GERD) 91
Barrett's Esophagus 91
Mallory - Weiss Tear 92
Achalasia 92
Diffuse Esophageal Spasm 92
Nutcracker Esophagus 93
Esophageal Strictures 93
Esophageal (Schatzki) Ring 93
Esophageal Varices 94
Boerhaave's Syndrome 94
Zenker Diverticulum 94
Gastric Disorders 95
Gastritis 95
Peptic Ulcer Disease (PUD) 95
H. Pylori 95
Zollinger - Ellison Syndrome 96
Pyloric Stenosis 96
Biliary Disorders 97
Cholecystitis 97
Cholelithiasis 97
Choledocholithiasis 97
Acute (Ascending) Cholangitis 98
Primary Sclerosing Cholangitis 98
Hepatitis A 99
Hepatitis B 99
Hepatitis C 99
Hepatitis D 100
Hepatitis E 100
Autoimmune Hepatitis 100
Cirrhosis 101
Fatty Liver Disease 101
Budd - Chiari Syndrome 102
Gilbert's Syndrome 102
Primary Biliary Cholangitis 102
Pancreatic & Small Bowel Disorders 103
Pancreatitis 103
Acute 103
Appendicitis 103
Bowel Obstruction 104
Small 104
Large 104
Paralytic Ileus (Ogilvie's) 104
Ischemic Colitis 105
Volvulus 105
Colorectal Disorders 106
Anorectal Abscess 106
Anorectal Fistula 106
Anal Fissure 106
Constipation 107
Hemorrhoids 107
Colon Polyps 108
Lynch Syndrome 108
Peutz - Jeghers Syndrome 108
Diverticulosis 109
Diverticulitis 109
Intussusception 109
Toxic Megacolon 110
Irritable Bowel Syndrome (IBS) 110
Inflammatory Bowel Disease 111
Ulcerative Colitis 111
Crohn's Disease 111
GI Neoplasms 112
Esophageal Cancer 112

Adenocarcinoma 112
Squamous Cell Carcinoma 113
Stomach Cancer 113
Hepatocellular Carcinoma 113
Pancreatic Cancer 114
Colon Cancer 114
Carcinoid Syndrome 115
Metabolic Disorders & Misc. GI 116
Phenylketonuria (PKU) 116
Celiac Sprue 116
Wilson's Disease 117
Lactose Intolerance 117
Hernias 118
Indirect Inguinal Hernia 118
Direct Inguinal Hernia 118
Hiatal/Diaphragmatic Hernia 118
Epigastric/Ventral Hernia 119
Umbilical Hernia 119
Femoral Hernia 119
Diarrhea 120
Infectious Diarrhea 120
S. Aureus 120
Vibro 120
C. Perifringes 120
Shigella 120
Salmonella 120
Rotavirus 121
Norovirus 121
Giardia 121
Traveler's Diarrhea 121
Typhoid 121
Cholera 121
C. Difficile 122
Bariatric Surgeries 122
Dumping Syndrome 122
Vitamin Deficiencies 123
A, B1, B2, B3, B6, B12, C, D, E, K 123
Vitamin Excess 124
A, B3, C, D 124

Pilonidal Disease: In Derm
G6PD Deficiency: In Heme
Hemochromatosis: In Heme

Musculoskeletal/Rheumatology 132
Elbow & Forearm 134
Elbow Dislocation 134
Olecranon Bursitis 134
Biceps Tendonitis 135
Biceps Tendon Rupture 135
Medial Epicondylitis 135
Lateral Epicondylitis 135
Elbow & Supracondylar Fractures 136
Radial Head Fracture 136
Nightstick Fracture 137
Monteggia Fracture 137
Galeazzi Fracture 138
Cubital Tunnel Syndrome 138
Disorders of the Wrist & Hand 139
Wrist & Hand 139
Scaphoid Fracture 140
Boxer's Fracture 140
Bennett Fracture 141
Rolando Fracture 141
De Quervain's Tenosynovitis 142
Gamekeeper's Thumb 142
Carpal Tunnel Syndrome 143
Colles' Fracture 143
Smith's Fracture 143
Mallet Finger 144
Boutonniere Deformity 144
Swan Neck Deformity 144
Trigger Finger 145
Dupuytren's Contracture 145
Felon 145
Paronychia 146
Finger Fracture 146
Flexor Tenosynovitis 146
Shoulder 147
Shoulder Fracture 149
Bankart Lesion 149
Hills - Sachs Lesion 149
Shoulder Dislocation 150
Clavicle Fracture 150
Acromioclavicular (AC) Joint Injury 151
SLAP Lesion 151
Rotator Cuff Tendinopathy 152
Supraspinatus Tear 152

- Shoulder Impingement Syndrome 152
- Thoracic Outlet Syndrome 152
- Subscapularis Tear 153
- Frozen Shoulder/Adhesive Capsulitis 153

Knee 154
- Patellofemoral Pain Syndrome 154

Ligament Injuries 155
- Anterior Cruciate Ligament (ACL) 155
- Posterior Cruciate Ligament (PCL) 155
- Medial Collateral Ligament (MCL) 155
- Lateral Collateral Ligament (LCL) 155
- Meniscus Tear 156
- Patellar Tendonitis 157
- Patellar/Quadriceps Tendon Rupture 157
- Patella Dislocation 158
- Patellar Fracture 158
- Baker's Cyst 158
- Tibial Plateau Fractures 159
- Femoral Condyle Fractures 159

Ankle & Foot 160
- Ankle Sprain 161
- Ankle Strain 161
- Syndesmotic Sprain 162
- Achilles Tendon Rupture 162
- Bunion (Hallux Valgus) 162
- Jones Fracture 163
- Pseudo - Jones Fracture 163
- Lisfranc Injury 164
- Plantar Fasciitis 164
- Morton's Neuroma 165
- Tarsal Tunnel Syndrome 165
- Pilon/Plafond Fracture 166
- Maisonneuve Fracture 166

Hip 167
- Avascular Necrosis of Hip 168
- Legg - Calve - Perthes Disease 168
- Hip Dislocation 169
- Hip Fracture 169
- Pelvic Fracture 170
- Iliotibial Band Syndrome 170

Spine Fractures 171
- Clay Shoveler's Fracture 171
- Hangman's Fracture 171
- Jefferson Fracture (C1) 171
- Odontoid Fracture (C2) 172
- Basilar Skull Fracture 172
- Atlantoaxial Dislocation 172

Back 173
- Ankylosing Spondylitis 174
- Back Pain/Strain 174
- Cauda Equina Syndrome 174
- Herniated Nucleus Pulposus 175
- Spinal Stenosis 175
- Kyphosis 176
- Brown - Séquard Syndrome 177
- Spondylosis 177
- Spondylolysis 177
- Spondylolisthesis 177
- Spinal Epidural Abscess 178
- Scoliosis 178

Other MSK Disorders 179
- Compartment Syndrome 179
- Osteoarthritis 179
- Osteoporosis 180
- Ganglion Cyst 180
- Rhabdomyolysis 181
- Paget's Disease 181
- Pectus Excavatum 182
- Pectus Carinatum 182

Bone Tumors 183
- Osteosarcoma 183
- Ewing Sarcoma 183
- Chondrosarcoma 183
- Osteochondroma 184
- Fibrosarcoma 184
- Osteoid Osteoma 184

Infectious MSK disorders 185
- Osteomyelitis 185
- Septic Arthritis 185

Rheumatologic MSK disorders 186
- Fibromyalgia 186
- Sjögren's Syndrome 186
- Systemic Lupus Erythematosus (SLE) 187
- Antiphospholipid Syndrome 187
- Scleroderma 188
- Polyarteritis Nodosa 189
- Rheumatoid Arthritis (RA) 189
- Polymyositis 190
- Dermatomyositis 190

- Polymyalgia Rheumatica (PMR) 191
- Reactive Arthritis (Reiter) 191
- Juvenile Idiopathic Arthritis 192
- Psoriatic Arthritis 192
- Seronegative Spondyloarthritis 192

Other Rheumatologic Conditions 193

- Gout 193
- Pseudogout 193
- Takayasu Arteritis 193
- Kawasaki Disease 194
- Granulomatosis with Polyangiitis (Wegener's) 194
- Eosinophilic Granulomatosis with Polyangiitis (Churg - Strauss) 195
- Microscopic Polyangiitis 195
- IgA Vasculitis (Henoch - Schönelien Purpura) 195

Rheumatologic Labs 196

EENT 203

Eye Disorders 203

- Blepharitis 203
- Orbital Floor Fracture (Blowout) 203
- Cataract 204
- Chalazion 204
- Hordeolum (Stye) 204
- Chemical Burns (Ocular) 205
- Conjunctivitis 205
  - Bacterial 205
  - Viral 205
  - Allergic 205
- Corneal Abrasion 206
- Corneal Ulcer (Keratitis) 206
  - Bacterial Keratitis 206
  - HSV Keratitis 206
- Ectropion 207
- Entropion 207
- Globe Rupture 207
- Glaucoma 208
  - Acute 208
  - Chronic 208
- Hyphema 208
- Macular Degeneration 209
- Optic Neuritis 209
- Orbital (Septal) Cellulitis 210
- Periorbital (Preseptal) Cellulitis 210
- Papilledema 210
- Pterygium 211
- Retinal Detachment 211
- Central Retinal Artery Occlusion 212
- Central Retinal Vein Occlusion 212
- Retinopathy 213
  - Diabetic (Non - Proliferative) 213
  - Diabetic (Proliferative) 213
  - Hypertensive 213
- Strabismus 214
- Uveitis 214
  - Anterior 214
  - Posterior 214
- Hyperopia 215
- Myopia 215
- Visual Pathway Defects 216

Ear Disorders 217

- Acute Otitis Media 217
- Chronic Otitis Media 217
- Mastoiditis 218
- Acute Otitis Externa 218
- Malignant Otitis Externa 218
- Acoustic Neuroma 219
- Cerumen Impaction 219
- Cholesteatoma 219
- Eustachian Tube Dysfunction 220
- Hearing Loss 220
  - Conductive 220
  - Sensorineural 220
- Auricular Hematoma 220
- Otosclerosis 221
- Tinnitus 221
- Tympanic Membrane Perforation 221
- Tympanosclerosis 221
- Vertigo 222
  - Peripheral 222
  - Central 222
- Benign Paroxysmal Positional Vertigo (BPPV) 223
- Ménière Disease 223
- Vestibular Neuritis 224
  - Labyrinthitis 224

Nose/Sinus Disorders 225

- Rhinosinusitis (Acute Sinusitis) 225
- Chronic Sinusitis 225
- Allergic Rhinitis 226
- Foreign Body 226

Nasal Polyps (Samter's Triad) 226
Epistaxis 227
Anterior 227
Posterior 227
Throat Disorders 228
Acute Pharyngitis/Tonsillitis 228
Viral Pharyngitis 228
Strep Pharyngitis 228
Aphthous Ulcer 229
Croup (Parainfluenza) 229
Epiglottitis 229
Laryngitis 230
Ludwig's Angina 230
Oral Candidiasis (Thrush) 230
Erythroplakia 231
Oral Leukoplakia 231
Oral Hairy Leukoplakia 231
Oral Lichen Planus 232
Peritonsillar Abscess 232
Retropharyngeal Abscess 232
Parotitis/Sialadenitis 233
Sialolithiasis 233
EENT Neoplasms 234
Nasopharyngeal Carcinomas 234

Herpes Simplex Virus 1: In ID

Bibliography

Images:

iStock. "Royalty-Free Stock Images, Photos and Pictures." iStock, 2021, https://www.istockphoto.com/.

Shutterstock. "Royalty-Free Stock Images, Photos, Vectors, Video, and Music." Shutterstock, 2021, https://www.shutterstock.com/.

Resources:

Epocrates. "Point of Care Medical Applications." Epocrates, 2021, https://www.epocrates.com/.

Wolters Kluwer. "Solutions for Professionals." Wolters Kluwer, 2021, https://www.wolterskluwer.com/.

Williams, Dwayne A,. *PANCE Prep Pearls V3.* Independently published (November 28, 2019)

National Commission on Certification of Physician Assistants. "PANCE Blueprint." NCCPA, 2021, https://www.nccpa.net/become-certified/pance-blueprint/.

The Diagnostic and Statistical Manual of Mental Disorders version 5

www.ingramcontent.com/pod-product-compliance
Lightning Source LLC
Chambersburg PA
CBHW041321210926
51847CB00002B/11